A LIFE WORTH
BREATHING

A LIFE WORTH BREATHING

A Yoga Master's Handbook of
Strength, Grace, and Healing

MAX STROM

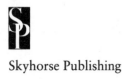

Skyhorse Publishing

Skyhorse Publishing books may be purchased in bulk at special discounts for sales promotion, corporate gifts, fund-raising, or educational purposes. Special editions can also be created to specifications. For details, contact the Special Sales Department, Skyhorse Publishing, 307 West 36th Street, 11th Floor, New York, NY 10018 or info@skyhorsepublishing.com.

Skyhorse® and Skyhorse Publishing® are registered trademarks of Skyhorse Publishing, Inc.®, a Delaware corporation.

Visit our website at www.skyhorsepublishing.com.

15 14 13 12 11 10

Library of Congress Cataloging-in-Publication Data is available on file.
ISBN: 978-1-61608-427-1

Printed in the United States of America

This book is dedicated to those who are on the path toward the light within, and to those who mark the way.

The Unnamable

There are times in these writings where the term *God* is used. Please feel unconstrained by this term, which is actually a symbol and not a name at all, and feel free to translate it to whatever name you prefer: Jesus, Adonai, Elohim, Allah, Yahweh, the Divine Mother, Vishnu, your Highest Power, etc. Most good people I know wouldn't mind being called by a different or inaccurate name, and God, being all merciful and the Lord of Love, is certainly vastly more merciful than any of us. So, I suspect that the God of love wouldn't mind if we called him/her/ it by a different name, even if potentially incorrect. So, if God doesn't mind, then why should we? There are so many things that God would prefer us to do with our time and energy, such as love and care for each other as instructed in all the major religious texts.

Friends, let us not quibble over what we name the unnamable; instead, let us concentrate instead on how we pronounce him/her/it with our very lives. God is in the essence of religious teachings, not in the details. As they say, "The devil is in the details."

Introduction

We can do more with our life. We all know it, we all wish for it, but just how to do it—that eludes us. As one man describes his life, "In the morning I can't wake up, in the day I am bored, in the evening I am tired, and at night I can't sleep." Even if we want to change, we're not sure which path to take, and if we do find our way, we are usually too emotionally wounded, physically unhealthy, or mentally stressed to take the steps we know would transform our desperate life into a meaningful one.

Most of us also long to change this troubled world, but the one thing we have the most influence over is the person looking back at us in the mirror every morning. We live in fear of terrorism, but in actuality, the most devastating terrorism comes from within as we continue to sabotage ourselves. A neglected body, chaotic mind, or wounded heart will prevent us from fulfilling our destiny as much as any outside enemy.

We know that we deserve and are meant to live an inspired life that rises above mere existence—but how?

FIRST: *Heal the body.* With the body revitalized, you can function at a higher level in all other aspects. Learn to govern the body so the body doesn't govern you.

Second: *Calm the mind.* The more still and clear your mind is, the better your decision-making process will be, allowing you to choose from wisdom rather than fear or desire.

Third: *Heal your heart, your emotions.* The more your heart is open and filled with joy and gratitude, the more you will enjoy life and be able to shine your light out into the world. The more light you shine into the world, the more you can help others with your very presence.

Change needs to occur simultaneously in all three aspects—body, mind, and emotions—resulting in a new state of being for which there is no price. You will begin to live a life you have always known you could live, a life with meaning, a life full of love, a life worth breathing.

The wisdom offered in this book integrates naturally with nearly all religious paths and philosophies because it does not attempt to replace them. Instead, it helps you embody your own highest ideal of life. It doesn't ask you to change your religion; it helps you to live your faith more fully. It does this partly by teaching universal principles of virtue that echo in the sacred texts of all the world's religions.

The primary intent is to learn to breathe the ultimate Source of Life, or Universal Intelligence—to merge with it, and to ultimately embody it. But what is the Source of Life? It is the Providence beyond names and words, beyond what our intellect can grasp, but what the heart knows intimately. People across the globe and across time have given this power various names, faces, and personalities, but we all know that the true experience of divinity is what we experience within. It is as if different people need different keys to unlock the same door. These keys, languages, and rituals open the mind and the heart and enable us to know reality beyond this world. For some it is a distant feeling of knowing and faith, while for others it's a blazing experience they can touch and breathe. But just as there are hundreds of names for the one sun that warms this earth, I invite you to seek the sun within you, and do so without imposing a name.

One of the essential practices of our time is hatha yoga, and it is sweeping across the world at an exponential speed. Why? One might ask, "How does this exotic workout have any meaningful impact on our happiness? On our relationships? Our careers?" The ultimate power of yoga lies beyond what the eyes can see. Hatha yoga, sometimes mistaken as simply a healthy form of exercise, is indeed partly a health regime, but good health comes as a side effect of a grander intent. Its purpose is to infuse our highest ideals (or spirituality) into everyday living, into our very bodies, wherein grace, harmony, and kindness become a way of life.

This book is not an attempt to elucidate one particular branch of yoga philosophy. Volumes of books have been written on the subject of yoga. In fact, one could spend a lifetime reading the vast ocean of books that have been written about the different forms of yoga, many of which contain conflicting philosophies. There is not just one form of yoga; in fact, there are entire cultures and dogmas that have sprung forth through the centuries as people have attempted to follow various paths of yoga.

This book moves respectfully beyond the cultures and dogmas of yoga, and instead concentrates on pure and practical techniques and exercises that will lead you into yourself. For all knowledge and wisdom resides within, and that is, finally, the purpose of yoga; to help us on our journey within. This work requires no Sanskrit knowledge, no chanting to deities or reciting of mantras. These things are not wrong, and are very helpful for many, but they also are not required to transform yourself.

The insights offered in this book are found not only in yoga, but also in the wisdom of the early Christians, in seminal Buddhism, Sufi philosophy, and Taoist Qi Gong. They are all branches of the same tree. When one looks at such teachings beyond the trappings of the cultures and religious institutions that claim to possess them, one will clearly see a thread that holds the necklace of religions together. It is this thread that will be revealed in this book. *The Kingdom of God is within you*—this is the chief lesson of so many teachers, from Jesus to Lao Tzu. They expound that within you is where the ultimate truth resides, and it is from the core of my heart that I received the message of this book.

To people who belong to a Christian church, I remind you that God was working miracles in this world and offering great teachings to humanity for thousands of years before the coming of Jesus of Nazareth; and did so across the globe, not just in the tiny area of ancient Judea. To exclude the illuminations God gave to man in other lands and on other continents would be like discarding the Old Testament and all of its inspired teachings. Great wisdom can be found in writings across the globe and across time.

All of the techniques and insights in this book are ultimately designed to help you to finally live a meaningful and joyful life, guided by the spirit within, and to accelerate your personal evolution.

In these times of religiously motivated wars and carnage, it is clear that we must reestablish the consciousness of unity, to see our similarities over our differences, to see the multifarious religions as we do different languages of different peoples. No matter what we call the sun, it will warm us just the same. To fight over names and regional customs was clearly not the intention of the great prophets of the world. This sort of religious-based violence indicates that what is desperately missing in our modern world is humility, for a humble person would never think of ridiculing another person's form of worship. A virtuous person sees the essence of religion and is tolerant of form. There is no need of any quarrel. We may not always be of one mind, but we can be of one heart. I have been guided from within to offer these teachings in friendship and brotherhood. May we all become teachers of peace, and teach in the only way possible: by example.

Acknowledgments

I extend my thanks to my editor Ann Treistman for her belief in this book and help improving it through the editing process.

Tony Lyons for his support.

The team at Skyhorse.

Andrea Barzvi at ICM for her steadfast and positive work.

Liz Delaney and Lori Snyder for their editing insights early on.

Also, thanks to my friends Carl Wright, James Courtney, and Ken Heitz for their encouragement to walk the path of my destiny so many years ago.

A special thanks to my friend Chris Silbermann for his encouragement and deep belief that this book would become a reality, and his help in making it so.

And my deepest gratitude to my wife, Stephanie Cate Strom, for her invaluable and wise insights, patience, and love.

My Beginnings

I was born in Santa Cruz, California, a twelve-pound baby with severe clubfoot. In fact, my feet didn't even look like feet, but rather curled toes sticking out from the ends of my legs with no visible heels at all. At four weeks old, the doctors plastered both my feet in casts in the hope that the casts would guide my feet straight as they grew. I was in plaster casts or braces for a considerable part of the first six years of my life. For an active and unusually large child, this was not ideal, but I learned to endure partial confinement and immobility for great lengths of time. In yoga we call this practice *tapas*, and it helped me to develop a high tolerance for pain and a deep patience toward discomfort. After the casts, braces, and two corrective surgeries, I was able to walk fairly well, but my feet were still abnormally shaped, three sizes different from one another, and not entirely mechanically sound.

As a very active boy, I seemed to have a knack for getting injured. I broke my right femur (thighbone) at age four, which demanded a cast from foot to hip. The result on my hips from all of the immobility was that by age five, even without the casts on, I was unable to sit cross-legged. I had almost no outward rotation of my hips at all. Another significant injury occurred at age ten when I fell from a tree, breaking my elbow. The break caused me to lose 40 percent of the use of that joint—not very auspicious for a future yoga practitioner.

These initial physical setbacks did not prevent me from developing into a healthy and strong young man. By high school, I was six-foot-four and a zealous football player. Even though I was an avid and aggressive athlete, I also became an inquisitive seeker, wanting to make sense of the world around me. It was this new introspection—along with a growing empathy for others—that made me feel remorse for the serious injuries I caused to my opponents on the field. This culminated during a game when I tackled a running back, head-on, and the boy was knocked unconscious. At first the audience cheered wildly, my coach shouted praise, and my teammates slapped my back enthusiastically, but after two minutes the boy hadn't awakened. The field grew quiet. After five minutes he was still unconscious and was taken away in an ambulance. I felt nauseated with the dread that he would never awaken again. I learned a little later that he was fine, but it left an indelible impression of the danger we all faced in the name of glory and testosterone. At the end of the season, I let the coaches know I wasn't coming back.

I was not raised in a religious or spiritual household. My father, a pragmatist and devout atheist, regarded the notion of a spiritual quest as useless superstition. My mother, a nature lover and early feminist, was mostly agnostic. My parents did their best to instill ethical values in me and to awaken my conscience—neither would stand for lying, stealing, or boasting—but the central messages they taught me about spiritual life, by my father especially, were clear and bleak:

> There is no God.
> We have no soul.
> Everything about religion and spirituality is childish superstition.
> When we die, life is over.

Therefore, I did not set foot into a church until the age of seven, when my family visited Paris. It was an unforgettable experience. The church was Notre Dame. My mother was a history teacher, so we visited the cathedral for its historical significance. The vastness and architectural beauty was incomparable to anything I had ever seen. I was absolutely dazzled by the mammoth cathedral, and my seven-year-old mind then assumed that this was what all churches must be like.

At about age fifteen I began spending a lot of time hiking in the beautiful countryside where I grew up. I enjoyed going camping by myself for several days at a time, relishing the extended periods of not speaking. Numerous sunset walks on trails near my home led to the spontaneous discovery of seated meditation on the hillsides. No one taught me to meditate; it just seemed like the most wonderful thing to do in the presence of Mother Nature's sunsets. Of course, I kept my meditations a secret from my parents.

Around this time, several mystical experiences completely changed the course of my life. They caused an urgent questioning of the reality I had been taught by my parents and society, resulting in an ardent imperative to understand the meaning of life. Among these experiences were prophetic dreams. Having grown up with no exposure to religion at all, prophetic dreams were something that I firmly believed were impossible and ridiculous, so when I began to experience them, they shook me to my core. I was in spiritual crisis and I needed to understand how the world worked: What was I? Is there a God? And if there was, what was it?

Finding no support or guidance from my parents—who were quite certain (incorrectly) that I was dabbling with hallucinogens—I began a passionate search for understanding. There was no wise, kind teacher to lead me, but my own spirit and intellect guided me to read, with spiritual voracity, any philosophical book or sacred text I could find.

By the time I was nineteen, I had studied Taoism, both modern and esoteric Christianity, Sufism, some Buddhism, and Greek philosophy, and I was diligently practicing meditation and Qi Gong. I began to see and understand the world differently, along with the possibilities of what it meant to be a human being. What I lacked in my search was a role model, a spiritual mentor who could offer me practical guidance along the way. I had found extraordinary teachings in books, but I was looking for people who embodied such teachings. I sought out and listened to many teachers and spiritual leaders along the way, but in my heart I felt that they were proselytizers, not teachers, and in some cases, charlatans. The lack of a guide eventually left me in a very lonely and isolated place. My eyes and mind had been opened, but my heart was sad. Like a penniless, hungry man standing outside of a bakery, I could see and smell the bread through the glass, but I couldn't eat it.

Over the next twelve years, my spiritual experiences lessened, and my searching was gradually eclipsed by an extreme sense of isolation, and this isolation needed a voice of expression. This came forth as a passion for music and writing, and I became immersed in two subsequent careers based in artistic expression; first, in music as a singer/songwriter in a West Coast rock band, and then in film, as a working screenwriter in Los Angeles.

My originally pure artistic intentions were gradually eroded by the reality of the entertainment world, and I eventually found myself living a life I never intended, immersed in a culture that was, for me, not conducive to developing a meaningful life. I experienced many of the pleasures of the world as my ego led me down its path of glory through artistic vision and a modicum of fame, and then finally to eventual financial bankruptcy and a psychological catharsis. I felt corrupted and distressed. I had a great deal of knowledge, but this knowledge did not fill my heart; it did not bring me joy or fulfillment. I was not living an authentic life, and I was fundamentally unhappy. I was thirty-four years old, and I was once again asking the same questions I had asked at age fifteen: Who am I? What is my true purpose in this life?

By Grace, it wasn't long before I was introduced to hatha yoga and my quest was reignited. Yoga came to me like an oasis in a harsh, barren desert. It came when I least expected it, and, like Grace usually does, it arrived when I needed it most.

My Introduction to Yoga

When I stumbled upon hatha yoga nearly two decades ago, I knew well what spiritual practice was, and I knew what exercise was—but I had never seen a system that combined the two, except for Qi Gong. My first real hatha yoga experience was at a new yoga center called Yoga

Works in Santa Monica, California. It was my thirty-fifth birthday, and a friend took me to class as a gift. Mistakenly, she took me to an intermediate/advanced class. I assumed that I wouldn't like it, and that was almost correct. I struggled, sweated a lot, almost vomited from exhaustion, and fell sound asleep at the end. It was fascinating and unlike anything I'd ever imagined, but what began to happen afterward was the truly extraordinary part: I found myself in a state of mild euphoria that lasted for nearly two days.

At my birthday party that night, my friends, not knowing about the class, commented that my energy was different. My dreams that night were vivid, and I awoke the next morning in a position I hadn't slept in since I was a child. Physically, I felt better than I had in many years. Something important had happened, and, most important, it had happened to more than just my body. Three days later I went back for more. Yoga was immediately a source of great relief to my body as it began to open and heal. Inspired, I soon started practicing four days a week.

Even at my increased rate of practice, I was still astounded at how little I could bend my body compared to others. I was so stiff it was at times embarrassing, as no posture came easily to me. But soon, I had a wonderful epiphany: I *was* the "stiffest" person in class, *and I may always be*. And for the first time in my life that became *okay*. I decided to give myself permission not to have to be the best or compete like I'd been trained to do in sports—compete until you win, or die trying. I knew it wasn't possible to win this time, and I would never excel at this, but I still loved it. So, I gave myself permission to be the stiff guy in the back row, the guy who was trying hard but was kind of embarrassing to watch. I just didn't care anymore, and it felt so good to me. This *allowing* felt so liberating, I believe it inadvertently accelerated my practice tenfold. By allowing myself to be a beginner, the pressure was off.

After a month of practicing I finally connected the dots and understood hatha yoga as an integral part of personal transformation. This made my practice noncompetitive and even joyful. It was amazing; I started to feel like plates of armor were being pulled off of me, creating a new sense of physical freedom. My joints were opening and my muscles were elongating, but I was also opening my stagnant energy channels and pulling open my heart center on a daily basis, especially through the breathing practice. I attribute much of my rapid transformation to learning how to breathe well early on. That is when things really started to move. Through the breathing practice I really *felt* the way I *thought*. The way my mind worked and the choices I started to make changed. This, I learned, is because as soon as your system for making choices changes, it changes the course of your life. From little decisions to big decisions, you begin to make them differently. Instead of going here, you go there. Instead of eating this, you choose that. Instead of befriending this person, you befriend that person, and so on. All those little decisions change the course of your life.

After about a year and a half of practicing six days a week, I'd sit outside the studio for a while on an old sofa. It was usually around sunset, and the light was often a gold and salmon glow. On one memorable evening in November, the air was quite cold, but I sat in peaceful serenity. I found myself totally content to sit quietly without the company of another, with nothing to say to anyone, regardless of the position of my body in terms of comfort or temperature. I had no appetite for anything. It wasn't that I was trying to curb my appetites; it was just that I found I didn't need as much stimulus to be content and happy. On this cold November evening, the implications of this came thundering into my mind.

If I have no appetite—it is because I am already full. If I have no desire to go anywhere—it is because I have already arrived.

I was experiencing a new sense of being, of completeness. The next thought that arrived was: If I could prolong this being/feeling by practicing regularly, I would need fewer and fewer things/activities/ social interaction/stimulation, because I simply wouldn't desire them. It became suddenly clear why or how the ascetics I had read about gave up the material world. Renunciation isn't deprivation; it is simply a state of continuous non-appetite—non-craving. I do not eat donuts—not because I deprive myself, but because I do not desire them. Simple.

The value I suddenly placed on my practice was astronomical. It's what could be described as drastically lowering one's overhead, causing windfall profits. In business, when one spends less, the result is more profit. My life/energy profit margin was skyrocketing because my desire/craving/grasping was radically diminishing. You could say that I was mostly "full," much of the time. This caused me to stop focusing on what I desired in life, since I was usually full, and instead focus on answering the question, "Who am I?" The distractions of craving/wanting were diminishing, so my ability to see was increasing. As I began to see who I truly was, I then tried to learn to manifest that. I committed myself to living what I called *an authentic life*, and I weighed the value of everything in this world against the value I had discovered within.

I had a renewed spiritual imperative, and I was determined to weed out any part of my life that I felt was not authentic or aligned in integrity. The practice affected me so deeply that my friends noticed the positive changes in both my body and behavior; however, most of them were still reluctant to attempt yoga themselves. They had the usual reasons: They did not have enough time, or it was too expensive. I explained that if I took the time for yoga each day, I found more meaning and happiness in the other hours of the day. As for being too expensive, I would reply that being unhappy and living in fear is expensive. Being a physical wreck is expensive. Lying sleepless at night wracked with worries is expensive. Destroying your relationships is expensive. Needing to take medications to function is far too expensive. These things cost you your life. In my eyes, yoga was the bargain of a lifetime.

As my vision burst open through yoga, it became a system of embodiment for all of my studies and experiences, both spiritually and philosophically. Finally, my heart learned what joy was, and I felt my spirit heal from within. Since then, my life has continued to grow toward the light, like a plant reaching toward the sun.

A LIFE WORTH
BREATHING

ONE

The Yoga Revolution

We live in a unique time in history, both promising and ominous. As technologies continue to develop at an unbelievably increasing speed, it seems mankind is not maturing nearly fast enough to adapt. And so we find ourselves in a global crisis. Billions of people now covet the industrial world's wealth and are replicating its system of modern consumerism as rapidly as possible. But what they are ignoring, perilously so, is the fact that as materially well off as the West is, we are also chronically living what Henry David Thoreau coined "a life of quiet desperation." In America alone, over 40 million people, rich by the rest of the world's standards, exist on antidepressants and antianxiety drugs, while over 80 million people use sleep aid drugs. And if the emerging nations obtain the wealth and technology they desire, it is likely they will discover the same shocking revelation that Americans have discovered: They are still not happy.

In the Western world we have more time-saving devices than any other culture in history, yet how many of us have any extra time to show for it? In America, we try to make sense of life where it is considered acceptable behavior to watch TV for four hours a day. (The average American watches four hours of television per day, which equals two months of nonstop TV watching per year.) So, then what has become of our collective nervous system? We don't have to look far to see the answer. Americans are depressed and stressed out. How could this be in the most materially rich country on earth?

What can be deduced from this is that our careers, cars, computers, and even our flat-screen TVs will not ultimately make us happy, healthy, or safe.

In contrast to our forward surge in technology, the direction of religion worldwide continues to careen backward to the Dark Ages, more tribal than transformative. From holy wars over holy lands to holy wars in our own minds, each religious camp is flying their gang colors. Each has determined that their own Messiah of love or Prophet of peace should be pronounced the absolute. And if you don't submit, these gangs will destroy you, despite clear instructions from their Prophet or Messiah to the contrary. Democracy and Christianity delivered in so-called smart bombs; Islam delivered in car bombs. As the world unifies economically, it is fragmenting and dividing culturally.

One of the great hopes in all this is that in the past decade there has been a huge upsurge in people embarking on self-examination. People are again asking the big question, "What is this life about?" And no matter how hard we may try to deny it, the answer we are left facing is a spiritual one. Because of this reawakening, yoga is sweeping across the globe at a dazzling speed. Many are turning to yoga not only to exercise, but also as an alternative to the experience of a spiritual gathering they cannot find in a church, synagogue, mosque, or on a Web site. The reason for this lies in the chief difference between religion and Western yoga: Yoga is usually offered in a nondogmatic format, which makes it inclusive as opposed to divisive. If one needs reminding of the perils of divisiveness, one need look no further than the morning newspaper; all family, tribal, state, national, and international warfare begins with the template of divisiveness. The lower mind first divides, then derides, and then destroys.

In my view, the reason for yoga's nondogmatic approach to healing and spirituality is that the first purveyors of yoga who came to America wanted to make it more accessible for Westerners, so they excluded much of the traditional spiritual components. What is fascinating is that even though their intention was probably self-serving, the unintended consequence was that students were led by the practice—without dogma—to a more pure spiritual experience. This is because yoga takes one's spiritual life and vitality into one's body, healing it while removing stress and pain. After a time, the drugs one may have depended on to battle depression, sleeplessness, and anxiety are thrown in the wastebasket. It seems evident that the exclusion of dogma is essential for a broad outreach into humanity and that is what yoga in the West has inadvertently done.

Because of its message of healing, unity, and a simpler life, yoga may be one of the great rays of hope for our future. Why? Because yoga is being embraced primarily by college-educated, upper-middle-class thinkers and businesspeople in positions of power—the very strata of society that has the power to make the changes this world so desperately needs.

In my own experience as a teacher of yoga, I witness many white-collar businesspeople park their $85,000 cars, turn off their cell phones, and walk into a yoga room in a courageous attempt to transform their bodies and emotional states without the use of pharmaceuticals. The transformation is powerful to observe. First, they begin to detoxify and de-stress the body, and then both the mind and body begin showing signs of renewed health. Then something they weren't expecting happens: One day, they experience a sense of calm, radiating *beingness*. This wondrous heart-opening consciousness triggers the profound realization that a ninety-minute, fifteen-dollar yoga class fulfills many of their essential needs, more than any of their other possessions they have worked like dogs to obtain. This life-changing insight compels them to reassess their very purpose in life: Who am I? Why am I? Where am I going?

It is my opinion that the shift we are witnessing is no less than a spontaneous, magnificent cultural/spiritual revolution. A new world culture is developing before our eyes at an astounding rate as yoga is being embraced primarily by motivated, college-educated, upper-middle-class thinkers and businesspeople in positions of power. This is no small thing, because yoga is exposing this powerful stratum of American society to radically nonmaterialistic and unifying philosophies rooted in the practice of kindness, honesty, and peace.

One of the seminal messages of yoga is that we do not need a "bunch of stuff" to make us happy; instead, yoga teaches that we already possess everything we need to be happy within ourselves. So, what we are seeing, perhaps, are the movers and shakers of modern society becoming the seekers of stillness and joy. The corporate powers do not understand this movement, as corporate ideals are often diametrically opposed to this philosophy. There is no way to sell things to a populace that already feels it has everything it needs. How can you market the philosophy of nonmaterialism? Pleasure you can sell; joy you cannot. Of course they try anyway, creating something now dubbed the Wellness Industry. But there will always be merchants outside the temples selling the doves to be sacrificed or the relics of saints to buy for worship; this seems to go with the territory.

The world at large could reap untold benefits as the core of the world's white-collar workforce becomes more concerned with opening their hearts than filling their wallets. Any yoga teacher in the world can attest that yoga is visibly de-stressing and healing countless people each day. This new wave of peace and tolerance can be felt rising, and not just in America; the wave has now stretched across the seas to Europe, the Far East, and even the Middle East. International power cities like Hong Kong, Tokyo, Beijing, Singapore, Berlin, London, Istanbul, and Tel Aviv all offer yoga classes in impressive yoga centers. Lives are being changed, relationships healed, and souls inspired to reach beyond themselves and into the possibility of a greater world through peace, nondogmatic spirituality, and a joyous, conscious life.

For what we seek is within, and in yoga, this is where we dive headfirst.

TWO

Our Situation

There is an old story of a simple farmer who overheard some merchants discussing the concept of lowering one's overhead in order to increase one's profit. While plowing his field the next day the farmer was struck with what he thought was an ingenious idea to lower his overhead in order to increase his meager profits. He decided that if he didn't have to feed his hardworking plow ox, he would reap considerably more profit. The farmer had heard of great saints who had given up food altogether and lived long lives, so, he planned to very gradually decrease the ox's food over a year's time until the ox learned to live on nothing but water. Almost a year later, the farmer's plan seemed to be working smoothly: The ox did the same amount of work while eating almost no food. It eventually worked for over a week without any food at all, and the plan seemed like an astonishing success, but then the ox unexpectedly fell over and died, foiling the farmer's plan. The farmer lamented to his friends about his bad luck; it was such a perfect idea and clearly had been working just as planned, if only his ox had lived to see the experiment through.

The farmer was somehow oblivious to the fact that the ox had died due to starvation.

This story illuminates the human condition—how we will fight to the end to prove that our ideas are right, our value system is best, and our likes and dislikes are the most supreme. The only problem is . . . we are not happy. Our cleverness, vanity, and intellectual certainty will often mask the clear fact that our life may be a disaster, yet we'll fight to the death asserting that everyone else should think and live as we do. "Everything was perfect till the ox died"—the ox being our spirit.

EXERCISE ---

Answer these questions:
Is your state of health less than optimal?
Do you feel that you are always seeking but never satisfied?
Do you tend to be depressed?
Do you sleep poorly at night?
Would you say that you have a stressful life?

Conclusion:
If you answered yes to two or more of these questions, it is time to implement a new strategy. We are in charge of our lives, and therefore must carefully examine our actions to make certain they are serving our fundamental needs and our highest ideals.

Do your actions and choices make you and your family happier, healthier, and more enlightened?

Albert Einstein once said, "The height of insanity is doing the same thing over and over again and expecting a different result."

Finding Our True Purpose

So many of us are dismayed because we cannot seem to find our destiny—our true purpose in this life. But in order to find our purpose, we must first have a sense of who we truly are, and this is often nearly impossible to achieve. We cannot see ourselves as others see us. Because much of our emotional infrastructure is invisible to us, we must seek help from the outside. The exercise below is simple, clear, and beyond valuable. If you have the courage to listen to the truth, it will exponentially accelerate your growth. Remember: In order to embody a new perspective, you must first discard your old perspective.

EXERCISE ---

Choose four or five people you respect and trust, and who respect and trust you—people who know you in many aspects of your life. For example: your mate, your employer, your best friends, a teacher, or a grandparent. The task at hand is to make an appointment to meet with each in private, one at a time, for the purpose of critiquing you. I advise you not to choose someone with whom you have an emotionally triggered relationship, such as a parent or sibling, as they may not see you as you are in the present, but may be stuck on their idea of who you were as a child.

-- •

Guidelines for Those Critiquing You

Bring a notepad, or, even better, record the sessions.

Begin with, "I'd like you to tell me what you feel my strengths are. Tell me what you think I am doing well. Tell me what my talents and gifts are as you see them. Tell me how you see me in this world in terms of my life's work—how I can be of most service to the world. Please speak of my strengths first, and then we will cover the areas where I could use some work."

Then afterward, "Now, I'd like for you to offer some suggestions on what I could do to improve. What are my weaknesses or blind spots? Are there ways that you see me sabotaging or deluding myself? What are your suggestions on how to remedy these issues?"

Guidelines for You

You must assure those critiquing you that you will not interrupt them or become defensive. You will listen well, and record the session or take notes so you don't forget any of the important details. If you don't understand something you can ask them to clarify, but you must never interrupt, disagree, argue, or explain why you do things the way you do. The point of this exercise is to discover the truth as they see it. By gathering this information from a group of people you will see common themes, and it will become clear what your strengths are, as well as where you are weak or deluded about yourself.

Example: If one person says you are not dependable, you will probably dismiss this as an inaccurate opinion because your friend is (in your view) perhaps too uptight or fixated on perfection. But if five friends tell you that you are not dependable, then you must take note and listen. It is no longer one person's opinion against yours; their assessment must be taken as fact, not opinion. You are, in fact, not dependable.

This works in the inverse as well.

Another example: If one person says you are a gifted artist and should pursue your art professionally, but you do not believe in yourself, you will probably dismiss this idea as a worthless opinion because your friend, in your view, doesn't really know anything about art. But if five friends tell you that you are a gifted artist and should pursue your art professionally, then again, it is no longer one opinion against yours; their assessment must be taken as fact, not opinion. You are, in fact, a gifted artist, and you should get used to the idea and stop wasting your talent.

This is one of the most powerful exercises you can do to see yourself as others see you, and to learn the truth that you may be hiding from. One of the wonderful things about this exercise is how empowered you will feel afterward. It is so important to have your strengths articulated by others, to hear how and why you are respected; after this, hearing about your weaknesses isn't as bad as it sounds. This knowledge is worth more than gold, for if we fail in this life, it is usually our own doing.

In my own experience doing this exercise, I was stunned to learn that others saw me as a natural teacher, for I did not see myself this way at all. It was only from the insistent encouragement of a few of my friends that I began teaching yoga classes. If I hadn't done this exercise, I may never have found my calling. The exercise illuminates you, holds a lamp up to your face and says, This is who you are, who you have been. With this new knowledge you can finally learn what direction to walk in—and when you walk forward with true knowledge of your strengths and weakness, you will not fail.

Special Note

This exercise is so frightening for some people that they will never do it; this is because they don't want to know these truths, or because they are frightened the exercise will cause rifts in their relationships.

On the contrary, I have found that this exercise strengthens relationships because each friend you ask to help you is being offered a great honor. The exercise tells them that they are highly respected and trusted by you. They feel more seen and heard by you and will be grateful for it.

I did not create this exercise; it was passed along to me by a friend who asked me to critique him. I have since gone through the process myself, developed it further, and have passed it along to many others. Everyone I know who has done the exercise has found it to be of great benefit, as long as the steps listed above are followed closely.

Know thyself.
—Inscribed on the Temple of Apollo at Delphi

THREE

The Three Pillars of Transformation

We deserve and are ultimately destined to live an inspired life that rises above mere existence. So, why do so many fail at finding true happiness and fulfillment?

Here is an ancient analogy that vividly depicts the plight of the average person. Imagine a carriage in terrible disrepair, while the horses that pull it are half-wild. The driver is distracted and unfocused, and the passenger and owner of the carriage is a king or queen, who is asleep, dreaming he/she is a peasant.

The broken carriage represents our body, the wild horses represent our emotions, the distracted driver represents our mind, and the sleeping passenger represents our soul. Nearly all of our problems stem from chaos in one or more of these parts of ourselves. Our relationship issues, financial issues, health issues, and quality of life are largely determined by our degree of vitality and harmony in these three aspects.

So, what we need to do is:

- Repair the coach (the body)
- Train the horses (the emotions)
- Sober and focus the driver (the mind)

The result of this work is to reawaken the soul, represented by the sleeping passenger. The soul then remembers who and what he/she is and can begin to live a life fulfilled, a life worth breathing. This is the aim of this work.

The Three Pillars represent a system of self-development within these centers: mental, emotional, and physical. They are not physical centers, but aspects, or inherent personality preferences: how one thinks and what one is drawn to on a broad scale. Each person is mostly focalized in one of the three primary centers.

Archetypal Examples:

> Mental—mathematician, scientist, engineer
> Emotional—artist, musician, minister
> Physical—athlete, dancer, carpenter

Each of us tends to be focalized in one of these centers and underdeveloped in the other two.

Example: Imagine a nonphysical intellectual, awkward in his feelings and in expressing emotion. This caricature depicts a type who is heavily lopsided in the mental center. While perhaps excelling in intellectual affairs and earning a good living, this type will often languish in personal relationships and health issues, ultimately feeling unfulfilled and desperately lonely.

Most of us seek and defend a lifestyle that reinforces and nurtures our type, and can tend to avoid and even ridicule the activities of other types. This is true even among spiritual seekers; all three of these dispositions live in imbalance.

Mental

It is common to see mental seekers who are on a spiritual path look down on physical exercise and dismiss it, attracted instead to scholarly pursuits and meditation. You might study sacred writings every day, even in their original, ancient language. But due to your cerebral nature, you suffer in personal relationships because of a stunted ability to articulate, express, and react to emotions. Or perhaps you meditate for an hour a day for a decade or more but because of poor posture in your sitting practice, and lack of exercise, you endure chronic pain in your lower back and knees.

Emotional

The seeker who is emotionally centered tends to turn to prayer, sacred music, and art. You may be drawn to spiritual poetry or chanting. You are often someone who is not motivated to exercise and may also suffer from food addictions due to your sensual nature. You are often not grounded and can be unreliable. Forty percent of Americans do not exercise at all, and not so coincidentally, the largest industry in the country is the health-care industry. Emotionally centered seekers can also tend toward unreasoning zeal or blind trust in spiritual leaders, even fanaticism.

Physical

Then there are those who are attracted to hatha yoga as an ultimate physical discipline which you believe will bring about a complete spiritual awakening. You often avoid emotional work or mental disciplines such as meditation as meaningless theory. Although the most physically fit of the three groups, you often display a restless nature, which results in problems with sleeplessness, anger management, anxiety, grinding teeth at night, etc. You often turn to substances to unwind.

Each one of us, although innately focused in one of these three centers, can still be quite powerful in a second center. For example, a brilliant scientist may also be a star athlete. More rarely, a very few excel in all three centers. When someone achieves this, there seems to be almost no limit to his or her capabilities. These extraordinary people are sometimes referred to as Renaissance men and women, such as Leonardo da Vinci or Hildegard von Bingen, and are the most balanced and integrated among us.

The Three Pillars of Transformation offers a system of integration that brings into balance all three centers. This requires us to develop strength where we are weak and flexibility or openness where we are congested—in body, mind, and emotions. As long as we are imbalanced, our lives and our spiritual path will be hindered by our own nature.

When I was the director of Sacred Movement Yoga in Los Angeles, California, we often hosted luminaries from a variety of spiritual lineages. We had leaders from various branches of Buddhism, Sufism, and, of course, hatha yoga. On the evenings of the events I would watch as over a hundred people would file in to be in the presence of these excellent and rare teachers. It was most interesting to notice certain commonalities in the posture, level of bodily health, and mannerisms of the audiences of these different lineages.

For example, the Buddhist audiences seemed calm and quiet. Their discipline of meditation was apparent, as they were able to sit quietly on the floor for long periods of time. But also, as a whole, they tended to be subdued and aloof. Physically, their bodies seemed inflexible, even hardened, with a slouching posture. Those over forty years old revealed overall poor health.

The yoga students tended to have excellent posture and excellent health, but were more restless and less well-mannered than the Buddhists. The yogis could sit without discomfort, but because their minds were restless, this caused their bodies to fidget more. Their minds were not as disciplined as their bodies.

The Sufis appeared noticeably more joyful and friendly than the yogis or Buddhists. But the Sufis seemed to be the most restless of the three groups, and like the Buddhists, they were not in optimal health. Many had trouble sitting on the floor at all and required chairs.

It was clear to me that these three branches of spirituality have much to learn from each other. What was also clear is how important yoga is to enable and empower our other practices: breathing, meditation, rituals, and daily life itself.

Example #1: It could be that you are an intellectual who hates exercising. So, the therapy for you would be to exercise. The fear of the ego is that exercise will make you feel weak and awkward, but after a short time the converse is true: It will make you more whole, and therefore stronger and healthier. Becoming stronger and healthier will make you happier, lengthen the duration and quality of your life, and even improve your mental facility. Without health we are (or will be) in a perpetual state of suffering.

If it is within your power to heal, then you should make all effort to do so. If your mind is a jet engine but your body is a run-down 1969 Volkswagen bus, then the jet engine will be unable to make you fly.

Example #2: Perhaps you identify yourself with a spiritual group or religion, but in actuality, you have never thoroughly studied the book espousing your religion. You "skimmed it." Nevertheless, you are certain that every word in it is true and you are considered a bit militant when discussing your views. The fear of the ego is that questioning the teachings you have adopted, thinking them through in a logical way, will make you feel frightened and lost, but after a short time the converse is true: Knowledge gives you power, and it will make you more secure, and therefore less defensive or reactive.

Example #3: Perhaps you practice yoga on the mat for two hours a day, six days a week, but you avoid practicing breathing or meditation. The first makes you feel vulnerable, and the second makes you feel restless. You realize you are addicted to movement as a way to process feelings and thoughts, but perhaps you also use movement to escape from some feelings as well. Dedicating yourself to a meaningful breathing practice may be just the tool for you to learn more about your hidden emotions, and to learn to be still. Processing the hidden emotions may bring you more inner peace and end the chronic restlessness. This stillness will allow you to finally meditate without disturbance.

HATHA YOGA is a spiritual path and branch of yoga that focuses on attaining mastery over the physical body, emotions, and mind. It is based on ancient teachings primarily rooted in Tantra, and its purpose is to help people escape the cycle of suffering, death, and rebirth, and to achieve *Moksha*. *Moksha* can be described as the ultimate Liberation from all worldly existence and total God realization. Common hatha yoga practices include postures, breathing exercises, meditation, ethical conduct, and the study of scriptures.

BUDDHISM is a spiritual path based on teachings attributed to Siddhartha Gautama, commonly known as the Buddha, or "the awakened one." Followers recognize him as an awakened teacher who shared his insights to help people escape the cycle of suffering, death, and rebirth, and to achieve nirvana. *Nirvana* can be described as peace with the world, free from craving, anger, and other negative states, and free from further states of death/rebirth. Some scholars consider Buddhism a branch of yoga. Common Buddhist practices include ethical conduct, meditation, mindfulness, and the study of scriptures.

SUFISM is often understood to be the mystical dimension of Islam, but many scholars believe that it predates Islam and even Christianity, and was born from the desert fathers from Central Asia. Classical Sufi scholars have defined Sufism as "a science whose objective is the reparation of the heart and turning it away from all else but God." In Sufi poetry, God is often referred to as "The Friend," or "The Beloved." Rumi, the thirteenth-century mystic/poet, is the most well-known of the Sufi saints. Common Sufi practices include ethical conduct, meditation, breathing exercises, prayers, and *Zikar,* or remembrance gatherings.

TAOISM is a spiritual path of Chinese origin that focuses on attaining self-mastery along with cultivating a close relationship with nature and the universe. The most important Taoist text is the *Tao Te Ching* ("The Way and Its Power"), written by Lao Tzu. Related to the Hermetic maxim of "As above, so below," Taoism teaches that man may gain knowledge of the universe by understanding himself. Taoism has had a significant impact on North American culture in areas of acupuncture, herbalism, and internal martial arts. Common Taoist practices include breath-initiated movement (Qi Gong), meditation, simplicity, ethics, and scholarly study.

FOUR

The First Pillar—The Mind

The Storm in Your Mind

It is the storm in your mind—the mental stress, negativity, and endless inner monologue—that causes so much of your emotional suffering and ill health. It is by teaching your intellect to become quiet, and learning to be still, that you can become happier, healthier, and more emotionally stable. Constant lurching into the future or dwelling on past events robs you of the present. True joy is experienced only in the present, so you have to be present to experience it.

Have you ever wondered why you cannot remember most of your life? It is because you weren't really there. You were hallucinating about the past or future so your consciousness missed the present. Why would you remember what you didn't experience? We live in a "greatest hits"—or "darkest hits"—of memory consciousness, and although many of our memories are negative, we replay them again and again. Each time we replay negative memories, we relive the emotions, perhaps even reliving a trauma.

Because they do not truly understand these concepts, many teach the need for a positive outlook as the solution to this problem; however, positive thinking alone is not enough, as our minds are so easily affected by external negative stimuli. For example, you can be in a very positive state but then be triggered into an argument in a mere moment from one wrong word. You must learn to achieve inner stillness, regardless of the outer circumstances. It is only when you can still the storm in your mind that you can unify mind, body, and emotions. Surrendering to stillness is an essential state of mind that the saints and mystics consider essential in order to know themselves, to develop consciousness, or to merge with God.

When the mind is still, the heart—our emotional center—is unencumbered, and when the heart is unencumbered, we feel joy, contentment, and peace. And then, instead of absorbing the world's chaos into us, more and more we can bring this stillness out into the world. Only after the storm is brought to stillness can we act from our highest Self, or soul, and not from the lower mind of craving, fearing, and so forth.

Be still, and know that I am God.
—Psalm 46:10

No thought, no action, no movement, total stillness: only
thus can one manifest the true nature and law of things
from within and unconsciously, and at last become one
with heaven and earth.
—Lao Tzu

Learn to be silent. Let your quiet mind listen, and absorb.
—Pythagoras

Those who have attained the summit of union with the
Lord, the path is stillness and peace.
—Bhagavad Gita

Peace comes from within. Do not seek it without.
—The Buddha

Your mind can stay turbulent and overstimulated for such a long time that you begin to believe this is how your mind is meant to be. Some people even feel afraid to slow it down, fearing they will lose their sharpness, though we all long for inner peace. Because of this, many of us have tried to sit in meditation only to find it a hopelessly futile experience, giving it up forever. We sit and try to get our minds to stop and feel like we're just sitting in the dark with nothing to do. This is because we try to calm our overstimulated minds but we have no idea how to do it, so we just sit with our eyes closed and our minds just as busy and fraught with turmoil as they were before.

Your natural state is alert stillness, so to relearn or remember how to achieve it is not as difficult as you might imagine. Remember when you were a child and you would go outside and stand with your arms out and then spin around and around until you got so dizzy you would fall over laughing? Then you would lie on your back and watch the world spinning around. Well, this is similar to what it may be like when you first try to sit in meditation: The body stops but the busy mind keeps going, spinning around.

In this section we will look at several aspects of the mind, concluding with how to bring the mind to stillness, and, more importantly, "why?"

SAINT (N): a person of great spirituality, virtue, or benevolence; one who touches the inner lives of others.

MYSTIC (N): a person who believes that spiritual realization of truth is beyond the intellect, and one who seeks conscious awareness of, or communion with, the ultimate truth, or God, through direct experience, intuition, or insight.

The Power of Intention

Our life is shaped by our mind; we become what we think.
—The Buddha

Nothing happens in the mind that doesn't happen in the body. They are one. The body is not the container of the mind; it is actually the mind that manifests the body. It could be called an extension of the mind. The body is like the yolk of an egg, the egg being the mind. When we direct our mind and heart in one direction, it gives our actions great power. This direction, or focus, is called our *intention*.

Example: Imagine seeing two people greeting each other with a hug. An insincere embrace and a sincere one can look very similar to the spectator, but to the recipient of the hug, the difference is vast. Now, during your yoga practice, if your chief intention is to heal the heart, open it to a higher power, calm your busy mind, and become healthier in the process, the result will be profoundly different from the person grunting through a yoga class to become slimmer and acquire firmer buttocks. Both mind-sets will achieve the physical benefit, but only one will transform your inner life.

If practicing postures until we are super strong and flexible were enough to make us into masters of life, then people would be flocking to the athletes in Cirque du Soleil to seek spiritual advice, as almost no one is more advanced in gymnastics than they. They are the cream of the crop of world-class gymnastic artists; compared with them, we are just playing in the sandbox. But are the Cirque du Soleil gymnasts known for having attained spiritual enlightenment? In most cases, probably not. My point here is that if these other world-class athletes haven't achieved enlightenment at their supreme level of physical ability, then obviously it's not just mastery of physical poses that leads to enlightenment. Postures alone do not necessarily transform us spiritually, unless one is driven by an intention to transform inwardly—a God-Intent.

> Remember, hydrogen and oxygen, depending on how they
> are mixed together, can produce either fire or water.
> —Vivekananda

Like the quote above, practice of postures—depending on how it is mixed together with intention and breath—can produce either "just exercise" or can help to revolutionize your life.

Now, there are some people on a spiritual quest who believe that any practice which involves the body is just another form of materialism. This is a perspective that is based in misunderstanding. I have met many people in their later years who have had dedicated spiritual practices but have disregarded the practice of yoga as unimportant, only to be plagued with ill health from a sedentary life and back and knee problems from lengthy meditations. They find themselves in physically disastrous shape in their old age. The vehicle we travel in must be kept in order, or travel becomes difficult, then painful, and then impossible.

How Intention Works

There is an old saying: "They say if you aim at nothing you're sure to hit it." Using the power of intention must not be underestimated. Once the conscious mind and our conscious heart align to a single purpose, the deeper mind—what some call the *subconscious,* begins supporting that vision. The subconscious begins filtering how you see the world.

Let us use a simple example. Remember the last time you purchased a car? Let's say you decided on buying a silver Prius. As soon as the Prius became your object of desire, your mind began to shift. When you went into town or onto the freeway, your mind began to seek out the image of the Prius, and you began to see them everywhere. Especially silver ones. And what's equally important is that the mind also starts to filter out most other cars. You saw Priuses all over town, whereas the person sitting next to you in your car may have decided to buy a different car, and he/she didn't notice the Prius at all, but instead saw the car that they desired.

Obviously, this phenomenon of the mind doesn't only apply to purchasing automobiles; it applies to everything. When you go to your local mall and people watch, your mind filter is in action there as well. If you are a clothing designer by trade, you will notice what people are wearing. If you are a dentist you will notice people's teeth. A jeweler will notice jewelry. If you are single and looking for a partner, of course your eyes will notice people who appeal to your particular preferences and filter out practically everyone else.

For those of us on a spiritual path, this phenomenon of the mind is a key tool that will help to empower us on our quest. For instance, the next time you go to the mall and people watch, what if you set your intention to look for a saint or spiritual master? (By these terms, I mean a person who is admired or venerated because of their virtue and profound kindness.) The mind would adapt to this request like any other. Then, instead of noticing people's shoes, clothes, teeth, or beauty, you would be looking at people in a new way. You would look past the outer clothing and even deeper than their skin. You would instead look into their eyes and at their countenance and bearing. You would begin to see into people's souls, and eventually you might even see a master.

We assume we would notice one now, but saints and masters are rarely seen by people with ordinary perception. If people with ordinary perception could see them, there would not be so many heartbreaking stories in history of great souls that were tortured to death or killed by angry mobs. Remember: When Jesus hung on the cross there were soldiers sitting nearby gambling, unfazed by the suffering of this great master nearby. If they had had eyes to see, this would not have been the case.

Today's masters and saints do not wear robes, and they do not have halos. We see them only if our souls are seeking them.

Upon rising each day, set your intention; whatever it is, visualize it. Each day at the beginning of your practice, close your eyes and focus on your intention. In other words, aim for something. Dedicate your practice to some transition you wish to have in your life, or perhaps some baggage you truly want to let go of.

Examples of what you may wish to release: Old resentment, grief, or addictions.

Examples of what you might aim for: inner calm, forgiveness, patience; perhaps complete union with the Godhead.

Your spirituality, however you define it, can be infused into your body so that you radiate who you are from your soul—and what you stand for in this world. Be clear that I am not talking about visualizing a stack of money or other such fantasies. I am referring to your life purpose, the vision of your soul's desire. Once you do this, your mind will begin to see the world in a way that supports that vision.

Prayer: *This morning may we all renew our intention. May we aim higher and believe in ourselves and each other. And let us all remember that each time we practice yoga, we help to heal not only ourselves but also our entire community. "May we be a breath of life to the body of humankind."*

The Ego-mind

The *ego-mind* could also be called the "false self," or "small self." It is a combination of our primary state of waking consciousness and our personality, but it believes that it is the body, intellect, passions, and name, and thinks it must fight for itself in the world. Put simply, the ego-mind is rooted in fear. It fears destruction of the body, reputation, and certainty. It also fears the awakening of the True Self, the soul, for the awakening of the soul would obliterate the ego-mind. It is like comparing the false idol to the true God. This is why the ego-mind fears the path of spiritual awakening and even mocks it.

When people say, "Anyone who believes that is an idiot," it is their ego-mind speaking. Or, "I hate it when . . ." Or, "My company is going to crush the competition . . ." These exclamations reveal a state of mind that is focused on survival, conquest, strong ambition, and aversions. Fear, hate, craving, etc., are born of the ego-mind. It thinks itself a king but is in fact a slave, for it reacts rather than acts. It reacts to desires of unknown origin, or reacts to aversions it doesn't understand. It fears stillness, for it associates thinking with being, so to stop thinking, it presumes, means death. This is the cause for hyperactivity and aversion to meditation. The ego-mind is a prisoner of itself. It will ignore logic, pretending it is following intuition when in fact it is being pulled along by the chains of compulsive emotions. Or, it may use logic as a justification for harmful behavior. The common thread is "I, Me, Mine."

The tyranny of the ego-mind is not unique in this world; rather, it is the most common state of consciousness and considered normal, although with closer inspection, what we call normal could arguably instead be called insane.

Many traditions state that man's essential error is the illusion that we are the ego-mind, known as *Maya* or *Samsara*. The ego-mind doesn't realize its intrinsic connection to all other beings and to the ultimate creative force in the universe.

The spiritual goal of Yoga, Buddhism, Sufism, and Christianity involves the dissolving of the ego, and the remembrance of (or awakening of) the soul from its sleepwalking state. (Remember the carriage allegory, with the sleeping passenger?) This awakening is known by many names, including Enlightenment, *Moksha*, Nirvana, being One with God, Universal Consciousness, and God realization. For example, in the *Bhagavad Gita* 2:71–72, it reads, "They are forever free who renounce all selfish desires and break away from the ego-cage of 'I,' 'me,' and 'mine' to be united with the Lord. This is the supreme state. Attain to this, and pass from death to immortality."

The ego will try and hijack your spiritual life, attempting once again to raise itself above all others. Your ego may tempt you to become a spiritual scholar and take pride in how many books you have read, or how many chants or poems you have memorized. But to proceed in this work, you must first understand that to acquire true spiritual knowledge—or in secular terms, to transform yourself on a deep and foundational level—you must first abandon the notion that spiritual knowledge is acquired through memorization or scholarly pursuits. It is not. To become an academic or scholar of spiritual knowledge is not the aim. *Information memorized* is not *knowledge integrated*. If memorization of spiritual data accomplished that aim, all those on the path with a photographic memory and above-average IQ would become illuminated. But this is not the case. It is a similar concept to the practice of hatha yoga postures: if the accomplishment of advanced yoga postures accomplished our aim, all those on the Olympic gymnastic teams would already be illuminated. This is also not true.

Whereas information is something you derive from books, *experiential knowledge* is derived from direct, personal experience. The mystic is one who makes direct contact with the divine source within, and it is from this experience that we can obtain experiential knowledge, as opposed to information that we are taught by others, or from books. Experiential knowledge is what we base our lives and our teachings on. It is all we have to go on when it comes down to it. Everything else can be fleeting and proven wrong; experiential knowledge is truly ours.

Anywhere but Here

The common state of the ego-mind is that it almost never wants to be in the same place the body is. "Anywhere but here," that's its motto. Again, this is the reason we don't remember most of our life, because we weren't truly present.

The ego-mind is very tricky, very cunning; it avoids being present and still. Watch how when you're extremely busy and distracted it will tell you, "I can't be still and peaceful now, there's too much to do. I'll be calm when things have quieted down." Then when you get into a peaceful situation, the ego will complain, "I can't stay present here, this is boring," and off it goes into the future, or to revisit past memories. Perhaps while practicing yoga, you'll find yourself in a posture thinking about your upcoming dinner, and then later you'll be at this dinner, and you'll be discussing your yoga class with your friends. "Anywhere but here . . ."

> We think very little of time present; we anticipate the
> future as being too slow, and with a view to hasten it
> onward, we recall the past to stay it as too swiftly gone.
> We are so thoughtless, that we thus wander through the
> hours which are not here, regardless only of the moment
> that is actually our own.
> —Blaise Pascal

In the context of your practice of yoga postures, the ego-mind has no problem injuring the body by pushing it too aggressively in the postures as it strives for its own glorification. It believes that becoming the most flexible or strongest is the very definition of happiness. But because it craves glory so intensely, it tends to ignore reality, like the fact that the body has limits. The ego-mind will push the body until it tears a muscle, or, worse yet, a ligament—yet once the body is hurt, the ego will take absolutely no blame for it. That is its nature. The ego isn't rooted in love and personal transformation, nor is it rooted in strength; it is rooted in fear. The ego tries to assert itself as powerful in its fear. In its insecurity, it tries to puff itself up in false grandeur. In its fear of its own destruction, it will strike out and harm or kill. In this way the ego-mind is at the root of complicated malevolent behavior.

Example: Let's say there is a woman, Alice, who is devoted to helping the poor. Out of her sincere love for the poor she devotes her days to their service at a homeless shelter. We would probably assume that Alice's demeanor would be loving and nurturing. But remember, the ego is insidious. So, Alice might be loving and nurturing to the poor, but her ego-mind might then hate anyone else who doesn't love the poor. She is so angry at the thought of someone being unkind to the homeless; she may obsess on it, and even churn in a slow-burning rage. Thus, Alice—who from a large heart loves the poor—is now angry and hostile toward those who don't. Then she's shocked to find out that people don't see her as a loving person; instead, they see her as an angry person. So, even though she is helping and protecting the poor for eight hours a day, her basic demeanor toward other adults projects anger and hostility.

We also see this sad phenomenon in "peace demonstrations," which often erupt into war-like riots. Remember, almost everyone who consciously does harm believes they are in the right, but the ego-mind thrives on the "ends justify the means" syndrome. We have recently seen this occurring on a national level in the so-called "war on terror." Because of America's fear of terrorists, who commit unthinkable acts of barbarism against civilians, our government—rooted in democratic values and the Bill of Rights—has itself been ensconced in torture controversies, with the White House and Pentagon claiming that we need to employ torture methods to protect ourselves from terrorists. The problem is, the people we assign to torture the "terrorists" are becoming ever more like them. And if we Americans are complicit in this, then we are equally as guilty. This is the final result of "the ends justify the means." This is a very common syndrome of human behavior: We become what we most fear.

If we are truly loving, we forgive those who are not. If we do not forgive those who aren't loving, then we become unloving. In other words, they will poison us with their unhappiness. Thinking we are the opposite of them, we actually become like them. This is what happened during the infamous Medieval Inquisition, when, in the name of God, religious leaders despised those who did not believe in their creed and branded them heretics, torturing them to death in vile and insanely cruel ways. The methods of the Inquisition rivaled the worst demons of the Inquisitors' imagined hell, all in the name of God, peace, and love. This is an extreme example, but the point is that this "Inquisitor" can be found within us all. Remember that we are all judged by what we believe, but we are judged far more by our actions. So, then, how do we, who see the paradox in others' violent actions, reconcile this in our minds? I believe this is where the teachings of a great teacher must come to the forefront: *Forgive them, for they know not what they do.*

The Present and Future Balance

Some of us have a very difficult time trying to learn to stay in the present moment, to keep the mind from fantasizing, planning, strategizing, and organizing the future. This is especially true for one whose career demands a great focus on the future. The answer is that one does not have to choose one way or the other as a permanent mind-set; the work is being able to focus on the future when it is necessary, and one of the many functions of your mind, but not the only function. And when one is not working, then you should bring the mind to stillness.

It is the same with the body; should it run or sit still? It depends on what is required in the moment. If it sits all the time it will die. If it runs from sunup to sundown it will also die. The art is learning how to bring yourself to the state of mind that best serves you in the moment. In our stress-laden society, more people need to learn to be still rather than grasping at the future. If you habitually ignore the meal before you, and focus on tomorrow's imagined meal, you will starve yourself to death. Similarly, if you ignore the hour before you and focus on an imagined future hour, you will be starved for fulfillment in your life.

When you are listening to someone speak to you—do that with 100 percent of your attention, as you practice conscious breathing.

When you are sitting down to meditate—do that 100 percent, as you practice conscious breathing.

When you are organizing your schedule—do that 100 percent, as you practice conscious breathing.

When it is required that you multitask—do that 100 percent, as you practice conscious breathing.

Train your mind not to run amok, even if it makes you money, or you lose control of your very life.

EXERCISE: --
Breathe Here Now . . .

In times of stress when you know you need to calm down . . . Breathe—do ocean breathing for three minutes (see page 112).

To become calm and balanced, you need to learn to stay aware of your body and breathe, just like when you practice postures.

Avoid the urge to needlessly multitask, but if you need to do so, try to remain present and aware while working. *It is the intention and degree of awareness that makes something useful or not.*

If you find yourself addictively dwelling on past experiences, remember that this moment is all you ever have. All moments are equal in their potential for growth and love. Whether or not a moment is precious is determined by the degree of consciousness and presence you bring to it. In this moment—now—do the best you can do. Create new and amazing memories

If you find yourself addictively dwelling on a fantasy future (it hasn't happened yet, so it *is* a fantasy), remember that you change the future only by your actions in the present. The future you are imagining will arrive as the present. If you habitually ignore the meal before you and focus on tomorrow's imagined meal, you will starve yourself to death. Similarly, if you habitually ignore the hour before you, and focus on an imagined time ahead, you will starve for fulfillment in your life.

-- •

Intellectual Humility

Humility is the elixir that invites harmony into the world,
for power without humility is tyranny. Physical beauty
without humility is ugliness. Material wealth without
humility is gluttony. The ego mistakenly sees humility
only as lack, so it turns away from it, while, in truth,
practicing humility brings balance and beauty to our
minds, hearts, and into the world itself.

It's an important step for the development of the mind to finally accept how little we really know, that the nature of the world is a paradox, and that our intellectual mind is incapable of understanding it all.

Opinions—they come and go. Look over your life and you will see how your own opinions have changed over the years. Things you were stridently sure of at age sixteen become laughable by age thirty. Once you accept this paradox, you will find that much more peace will reign in the nervous system because the intellect stops believing that it can ever understand and so it calms down. I'm not referring to blind faith—that's something different. What I'm talking about is the courage to experience something new without needing to label it.

Imagine a group of four friends on a night walk. A luminous object is spotted moving through the sky. One friend says, "Look, it's a flying saucer!" Another exclaims, "No, it's a weather balloon." Another believes it's an angel. And the final friend thinks, "I see something that I can't logically explain, but I accept that something there exists, and I also accept that I don't yet understand it." This last outlook leads to true learning, but requires a willingness to say "I don't know," to find peace in that and not fall into the childlike mind of "I don't know, therefore I'm going to get a bad grade, or I'm going to be laughed at by my peers, or I'm going to be considered dumb by my parents." All of these programs have been engrained in the shame of "I don't know."

If someone brings up a subject you know nothing about, don't nod your head as they speak, pretending you do know; be willing to say,

"You know, I have never heard about that. Tell me about it." Others will respect you for this and be more than happy to share their knowledge. Be honest and you will gain new knowledge every day; pretend to know and you will learn nothing. Learn to feel comfortable within the mystery we are surrounded by.

EXERCISE --
To learn to see more deeply, practice having no opinions for a time. Be willing to say, "I don't know." This "not-knowing" allows space for true knowing, because the intellect is not the center of spiritual knowledge and wisdom; this is the higher function of the heart within the heart.

--- •

The Power of Self-Discipline

It doesn't matter what you decide to do tomorrow as you go to sleep in your comfortable bed—what matters is what you do when the alarm clock goes off in the morning. It doesn't matter what kind of diet you decide to begin when your stomach is full—what matters is what you do when you're hungry and you are choosing what food to eat for your meal.

Think of how a magnifying glass can take a ray of sun, concentrate it, and burn a hole through something. Similarly, our magnifying glass is our discipline or will, and the ray of light is our intention. Our intention is magnified and concentrated until it burns away all obstacles.

Nearly two decades ago I met a professional writer who had served seven years of hard time in a maximum-security prison. He had been released from incarceration a few years before I met him, married a professional woman, and had become quite well paid as a screenwriter. One day a mutual friend took me to visit him at his home located in an affluent neighborhood. The house was quite upscale and decorated beautifully by his wife. The writer, however, didn't actually spend much time in this house. He wrote and often slept in his "room," as his wife referred to it. This room was located in the garage, which was austere and semidark. The cold cement floor was bare, and a stark industrial-style metal desk stood beside the simple bed. In short, it appeared that this man had re-created the prison cell in which he'd become accustomed to living. Although he was now technically a free man, internally, he had not freed himself.

Later, I learned that this tendency resides in us all. An alarming statistic reveals that nearly all lottery winners who lived in poverty before winning a multimillion-dollar jackpot were living in poverty again after only a few years, squandering their new fortune until their life was back to where it had been. This is a vivid example of the power of our inherent tendencies.

Clearly, we are indeed creatures of habit. Breaking old habits is by no means an easy feat. One look at the magazine stand in the grocery store and we are reminded how we all struggle with willpower as we see article after article on how to lose weight. Gaining control over our own eating habits can be a nearly impossible endeavor.

And this leads us to the question, What is a habit? It has been said that our most powerful habits, or *samskaras*, are the main part of our personality, carried over from one life to the next through reincarnation. In this line of thinking, then, our habits are a large part of our inherent infrastructure, part of the essence of our personality.

To transform ourselves it is critical to successfully "burn" these negative habits; not doing so can make our transformation next to impossible. It is like a hot air balloon: In order for it to float upward, one must first toss the sandbags overboard. Personal transformation is, among other things, a system of burning our unwanted habits and replacing them with habits that are helpful to our aim of spiritual realization.

Burning our unwanted habits is called *tapas* in Sanskrit—meaning putting forth extraordinary effort toward changing one's behavior, and even one's inherent tendencies. Simply put, it is a practice of exchanging old sabotaging habits for new transformational habits—exercising self-discipline. In the industrial world, we are known for working very hard and for very long hours. Because of this, we may feel we are no stranger to self-discipline. But this kind of effort alone cannot benefit the spirit. Spiritual benefit comes only when we focus extraordinary effort toward the intention of a spiritual result. Effort alone, even extreme effort, has no benefit unless the intention is for the awakening and transformation of the soul.

Here's an example: Think of a slave doomed to work in a rock quarry day after day, hammering stones to pieces in the hot sun. Throughout history, no one worked harder than the slaves used for manual labor. Unfortunately, their work led mostly to suffering, and had no internal benefit because it was done under threat of punishment and execution. The extreme effort put forth by the slaves was certainly not voluntary, and it usually was not done with the intention of spiritual benefit. The person who chooses to expend intense effort *voluntarily* gains inner strength because he or she is committed to both the work and the intention behind the work. Therefore, this person is driven by his or her own will, not the will of another.

Think of prisoners sentenced to life imprisonment. Their life is not so unlike a monk or nun who voluntarily commits to a solitary and austere life. The difference is, the prisoner is imprisoned against his will, whereas the monk feels an inner freedom because he is there by his own free will. There have been spiritual teachers who have taught just this lesson to prisoners. The message carried to them was, You are in here for the rest of your life; your daily conditions and life structure are not unlike a monk's, except that a monk chooses this life. So, you too can choose this life, and if you choose it, you will no longer be prisoners—you will become monks and you will be free.

One of the most potent ways of exchanging self-sabotaging habits for empowering new habits is to practice and cultivate self-discipline in a yoga practice at least four times per week. Unify postures, breathing, and focus; all three pillars. The benefits of practicing self-discipline in yoga are not confined to the yoga room. If you learn greater focus in your practice, your focus will also improve in your workplace. If you become more patient in your practice, you will become more patient in your relationships. If your manner becomes more kind in your practice, you will be kinder to all.

> If a regime of a ninety-minute yoga practice, four times per week, is not yet possible due to legitimate time constraints, follow the advice of the great yogi Theodore Roosevelt, who said: "Do what you can, with what you have, with where you are." Twenty minutes in the morning and evening is a great beginning, and you will see a difference in how you feel.

EXERCISE --

Cultivating Self-Discipline

To cultivate discipline, you must approach an unwanted physical habit—for example, eating too much sugar—with the constant axiom, "Will this action strengthen me or weaken me?"

If you still are struggling with taking the right action due to lack of resolve, courage, or strength, then ask yourself this question: "How can I transform this behavior to a new behavior that will empower me, and enjoy the process? How can I find joy in my new discipline?" Notice the key phrase in the previous sentence: *enjoy the process*. Instead of thinking *How can I get this done?*—try, *How can I transform this behavior and enjoy the process?* This is a totally different way of going after the same change. One seems like toil, while the other includes joy as a priority.

This mode of thinking will help you to unify the power of your emotions with your new imperative; then, your discipline will seem less like suffering and more like a joyous transformation—liberation rather than suffering. Digging a deep hole in the earth is drudgery; digging a tunnel out of a prison is inspiring. Remember: How we envision our actions, and how we verbalize our desires, unconsciously has a massive impact on the quality of our response.

-- •

Through the Eyes of Saints

What is the difference between a saint or spiritual master (think of Mother Teresa or Rumi) and an average person in this regard? A saint lives in the same world that we do, surrounded by the same problems. They witness the same suffering that we see, and are tempted by the same emotions of anger, resentment, fear, and grief. But saints seem strangely untroubled and joyful in this violent world. And so we scratch our heads and think, "How can such a caring person still be happy? Because it seems like if they really cared, then they would be upset by all the horror that goes on in the world, same as I am." So, then what is different about a saint's state of mind?

Here is an example: Imagine being in a car accident. You were on your way to somewhere nice for dinner, and then suddenly you're in a car accident, and now you're lying on the side of the road, bleeding through torn clothing. You're scared and in pain. And when the ambulance comes, the last thing you want is for the paramedic to get out of the ambulance, take one look at you, make a horrified face, and shout, "Oh, my God! What a mess! You don't have a chance!"

What you want is for them to do what they do: They smile, and say over and over again, "Everything is going to be okay. Don't worry; we'll take care of you. Everything is going to be okay. We've got it—don't worry."

I believe that's how saints are most of the time; they are in a state of nonattachment toward external circumstances, and they tell the world, "Don't worry, everything is going to be okay." And this is the state of mind that we reach for—breath by breath.

So, in our daily life, when we see tragedy, when we see evil, when we see suffering, we have two choices: We can take that suffering into us and become upset, or we can direct our joy and love and send it out into the suffering in order to heal it.

How to Transform a Hardwood Floor into a Feather Bed

After we go to yoga to heal our back, or to help us get out of a depression, then something else starts to happen, something inexplicable, and we begin to feel different. We focus more on our breathing practices and meditation, and we notice that we start to feel calmer and less reactive to others. We begin to see and feel the world differently.

I met a woman who used to have a serious drinking problem, and she said to me, "You know, when I stopped drinking, it's amazing how everybody straightened up and became nicer." It's like that with yoga—the more we do yoga, the more other people seem to become nicer. Have you ever thought about the last position in a yoga class, the final relaxation pose called *shavasana*? At the end of class we lie on a quarter-inch-thick rubber mat on a hardwood floor and fall sound asleep in three minutes. And we sleep well.

If we went to a hotel and they showed us a room with a bed consisting of a rubber mat on a hardwood floor, we'd walk out. But if we did our practice on that mat first, then the hardwood floor would be the most comfortable feather bed in the world, and we would fall sound asleep on the mat in less than three minutes. Did the floor change—or did we change? When we do our practice, the world we know appears to change, but of course it is not the world that has changed—we have changed. This is why when we practice, everybody else becomes nicer and the hardwood floor becomes a feather bed.

When you hear about monks and nuns who give up possessions, they're not renouncing anything. It is because of their practices that they no longer desire these things, as the desires simply drop away.

This is the great secret of the practice of the Three Pillars of Transformation: As we transform, the world around us appears to change, even bloom into a realm more like heaven. And this is why saints, or masters of life, seem so happy: They see the same world we do; it's just that they see the world though different eyes. We want less and give more, we notice beautiful hearts, and we are more forgiving of the mean-spirited. When we do our practice, it is as if we live in a different world with our hearts open wide.

As Jesus said in a Gnostic scripture, "The kingdom of heaven is spread upon the earth but men do not see it." When we do our practice, we begin to see heaven on earth.

EXERCISE --

During your yoga practice, while in postures, *breathe here now*—and still the mind. Bring your awareness to different areas of your body and imagine you are breathing in those areas.

Example: Imagine, and try to feel yourself breathe into your feet and out of your hands. Witness (hear, feel) your breath.

Witness the energy moving from your feet.

Witness your feet. Witness yourself witnessing.

Become a nonanalytical witness. This nonanalytical witness is your True Self. Now try and remain nonattached to the sensations of the body as long as you are safe in the pose.

Remain nonattached to how long you have been or will be in the pose.

Remain nonattached to if you are strong or weak, stiff or flexible in the pose. Remain nonattached to whether you look impressive or silly to others.

This is how to practice nonattachment in your hatha yoga practice. Doing this regularly has a cumulative effect. Compulsions drop off naturally with only a little effort. When the heart and mind are at peace, the desires of "clinging/grasping/wanting" begin to evaporate. You are present—the higher you.

After practice, sit quietly for a few minutes; experience this new awareness for a while, and feel your life without the constant distractions from the body.

-- •

Abandon asking for certain things to make you happy.
Why not just pray for happiness? Maybe God knows
better than we what would make us the happiest.

Happiness Is a Choice

One of the ways we sabotage ourselves from experiencing happiness is by demanding our happiness in a certain form, and this usually prevents us from getting it. For example, fame; if you are fixated on becoming a world-famous movie star and after years of determined struggle this never happens for you, you may be doomed to a life of constant disappointment, when in fact you may have many gifts laid before you that could bring you the deepest fulfillment. Being a movie star may not be your destiny in this life; you may be destined for something else. But many romanticize the struggle, ignoring healthy signs that they may actually be striving for something that ultimately is not in their best interest.

Nearly all of the great teachers lived by simple means, and fame did not come to them by seeking it; in fact, although many of them avoided the spotlight of society, fame came to them through their works and their very presence. Fame is usually a burden to those who are balanced people. It has been said that fame is far more difficult to overcome than failure.

Another example is consumerism: Our culture implores us to buy newer and better things, but research and intelligent observation show that our things do not bring us happiness. Money buys happiness only for those who lack the basic necessities of life.

One of the seminal lessons of a spiritual life is that ultimately, happiness is a choice regardless of your circumstances. The sages of yoga, Buddhism, Taoism, Sufism, Judaism, and Christianity all teach this. Happiness can be obtained even if you are picking crops, loading boxcars, or dwelling in prison.

Writer and teacher Viktor Frankl, a concentration camp survivor, said:

> *We who lived in concentration camps can remember the men who walked through the huts comforting others, giving away their last piece of bread. They may have been few in number, but they offer sufficient proof that everything can be taken from a man but one thing: the last of the human freedoms—to choose one's attitude in any given set of circumstances, to choose one's own way.*

As I have journeyed through my own life, I have realized that the most wonderful and meaningful moments are connected to my heart, and not the circumstances of the day. As I look back though the past, all of my most powerful memories are connected to either spiritual epiphanies or to love, the people I was interconnected with. The big "goals" that I set for myself as a young man fade from my memory like they were mirages, meaning less and less as time went on. True quality of life has always been determined, whether I knew it or not, by the degree of my own inner peace and my ability to love and accept love. Once I had practiced the Three Pillars for about a year, I became less interested in self-determined circumstances of pleasure, and more engaged and integrated with what was in and all around me. In other words, I began to let go of demanding happiness in a certain form, and began to let Providence determine the form, believing the Creator's vision of what is best for me is far superior to what is, by comparison, my own narrow view.

Remembrance

Consumer-based society trains us to search for our happiness outside of ourselves. We look for it everywhere except where it is—within. We unconsciously learn to disconnect from our breath, our body, and even our feelings. Go to nearly any business office and in the waiting room you'll find a stack of magazines to distract you. Step into your car and the stereo is soon on. Step back out of the car and the cell phone is up at your ear. And even at the gym, we watch TV as we cycle or run on the treadmill. This is called *disconnecting*, and when we create a habit of disconnecting from our breath, body, and feelings, we eventually find ourselves down a road we never intended to walk. We find that we have acquired habits exactly the opposite of what we need to have in order to improve our well-being. We begin to forget what living is. We forget that we are a soul within a body.

> HIGHER SELF—The higher Self is the Soul, your essential being, which is connected to the Ultimate Soul (or Spirit), the Divine Providence (or Godhead). Remember: you do not *have* a Soul; you *are* a Soul that has a body, a mind, and emotions.

Many sages from the Sufi tradition teach that in the world of spirit, we do not really learn about spirituality or God; we remember. In fact, many Sufi orders practice a spiritual ceremony called *Zikar*, which literally translates as "remembering," meaning to remember God, and who and what we truly are. It is a spiritual ceremony or act of devotion that often includes music, chanting, and breath-initiated movement. These teachings hold that deep inside, we have never actually forgotten who we are, but the memory has become buried under the unnatural concepts of our modern culture. They say that "we walk in the world with amnesia."

Yet nearly all of us have had remarkable moments when memory rises to the surface of our consciousness. Remember when you heard a song that you so deeply connected with, it sent shivers through your body? Or a place that, when you arrived, seemed familiar to you even though you had never been there before? Remember when you read a book and your hair stood on end as you said to yourself, "These are my words; I could have written this." These moments are glimpses into a deep remembrance or awareness of our higher Self and our inner life. They are glimpses into the connectedness of things; the more awake we become, the more familiar the world becomes, and the less we will fear it.

> *Realize that the power you seek is the power of your own soul. The peace you seek is there; the beloved you are seeking is there.*

Awakening from the Dream

Imagine that you're in a movie theater in the middle of a very good film an intense, passionate, profound, and riveting drama. Tears are running down your face as you sit completely absorbed, completely identified with this film. Your life is in this film. In this state of consciousness you are unaware of what's around you—your body, your past, your future; you're just there in the moment in this world that seems very, very real, and your emotions are heightened.

Now, imagine that suddenly the projector breaks down, and you suddenly you find yourself in darkness. What is your reaction? First of all, you would feel a shock to your emotions. Then you would probably become very upset because you've been forced out of the world of the film. You want to see how it's going to end, and how could this happen? You sit in the dark with waves of frustration and aggravation surging through you. The physical world of the theater is a numbing, dull experience compared to the living world of the film. You feel alone, isolated; you're almost desperate to have the movie come back on.

Then the lights are turned on; they can't fix the projector, and your film experience is over. When that happens, what do you discover? This drama you were so captivated by wasn't real. It was a movie—and, in fact, the person sitting next to you happens to be the love of your life. Sitting next to you, holding your hand, is someone you deeply love, a person of flesh and blood, whom you forgot was even there. You were so absorbed with the celluloid drama made up of flickering light and recorded sound, a story that never really happened except in the imagination of the filmmakers, that you forgot your own life, your own world, your reality. You forgot that your beloved was sitting right next to you, loving you. So, in a little while you settle down, you settle back into reality, you forget the movie, and once again, you are in the reality of your heart, your life.

I think this example is not far off from the journey of consciousness, from being totally identified with the hallucination of the collective reality, in contrast to witnessing the true reality.

So, as a metaphor, let us say that the first stage of waking up is to "shut off the projector" by getting on our mat and practicing yoga postures and conscious breathing. This slows down the mind more and more, almost to a stop.

The second step is to "turn on the light," to illuminate this dark room from the inside. This is experienced in meditation after we have slowed down the mind with postures and breathing practices. This is done by dissolving the ego-mind and by setting our intention to release "thinking." One way of doing this is to focus on opening the heart center. When we awaken our true consciousness, we can become aware of the Source of Life. The Sufis sometimes refer to this energy as "The Beloved," because when we feel this energy, it opens our heart and we feel immense love. This is "turning on the light."

Once the light turns on, we become aware of the presence—that The Beloved is with us. This is the experience of union with the source of life some call God. In yoga this experience is often called *samadhi*.

But what does *samadhi* have to do with your daily life? With washing your face, taking out the trash, or with driving to work? *Samadhi* will begin as something you occasionally experience in your meditation, but later you will experience it more frequently. Then you will be able to, at times, experience it at will even while involved with everyday tasks. Your senses will be heightened and your mind, vividly alert and profoundly present, and you will begin to affect the world like never before. Rather than *reacting* to your cravings and fear, you will finally *act* from your deepest Self.

Meditation—The Journey Within

> You should sit in meditation for twenty minutes a day—
> unless you're too busy; then you should sit for an hour.
> **—Old Zen adage**

It is nearly impossible to walk a spiritual path while the mind and emotions are in chaos and our bodies are weak and/or sickly. The aim of this book is to lead you into yourself, for it is within you that firsthand knowledge dwells. When you develop a meditation practice, you will begin to remember and have access to wisdom long buried. This wisdom will then guide you in the course of your destiny.

When your mind finally becomes quiet, the stunning thing that happens is, your heart opens. For you who do not understand what I mean by "heart opening," the nearest thing I can compare it to is how parents describe the feeling of looking into the eyes of their infant child and having their child look back at them and into their souls. This feeling that parents describe is the heart opening—when your eyes fill with tears and your heart feels like it could explode from so much love. Or the feeling in your chest when someone forgives you and you are reunited again and in their arms, and your heart swells with the feeling of everlasting gratitude. This is the kind of heart-opening phenomenon we speak of. So, when the mind quiets and the heart opens, change happens, and then, sometimes, Grace happens.

Here's an example: For the average Western mind, postures, movement, and conscious breathing are crucial to enable us to meditate. Imagine we are living in a nonmoving car that's covered in mud, but we aren't aware that we're in the car or that there's anything outside of the car because we can't see out; there's no context. All of the windows are caked with mud so we are not aware of anything except for what is inside this car. When we start practicing yoga postures and breathing practices, it's like cleaning the windshield. When we start cleaning the windshield, we realize there is a whole world out there that we weren't aware of. (Of course, instead of looking out, we're actually looking into our own being.)

Once you realize that you are in the car and there is someplace to go, now you begin to understand what all these instruments are for. They are meant to take you on a journey forward. The journey forward is the practice of meditation. You can think of the practice of postures and breathing as cleaning the windshield, and meditation as driving the car, traveling on the journey of your spiritual practice.

In the beginning stages, meditation can seem an inconvenience. Later on, you may feel like you could never go back to a life without meditation because it ceases to be a chore and instead becomes the more profound part of your daily life. Particularly during times of conflict, meditation can provide direct access to peace, to your most authentic Self, to spirit, to the Universal Consciousness—whatever you wish to name it. Somebody once said to me, "In times of adversity, meditation saves me, because during those times I have direct access."

Beginning to Meditate

Allow the mind to observe itself without the clutter of its thoughts. Allow the heart to observe itself without its wounds.

Sometimes when we first attempt meditation, because we don't understand what it is, we may feel like a young child sitting in a lonely room with our eyes closed. We read in meditation books to quiet the mind—just quiet the mind. Well, that sounds good, but *how* do you do it? For many it can feel stifling, boring, and ultimately pointless as our mind continues plaguing us with negative thoughts and worries.

We want to surpass the initial phase of restlessness described above as soon as possible. Here are a few suggestions for beginners at meditation:

Step One

Why don't we use the mind itself to solve the problem? Use the mind to trick itself into stillness. Instead of corralling the wild animal, we will ride the animal. The enemy will become our ally.

For instance, if when meditating your mind keeps lurching into the future toward the next planned destination, such as going to work, allow the mind to go to work in your imagination. But once you arrive in your workplace in your imagination, walk into your office and, in front of all your coworkers, sit on the floor and begin meditating. Or even on top of your desk. See the expressions on their faces. Then, if your mind travels somewhere else, the second you realize it, sit down in that dream world and meditate there. Continue this process and eventually the mind will give up and allow you to sit in peace.

Step Two

Next, we begin what is called a *heart-centered meditation*. Instead of focusing on clearing the mind, trying to be still, and trying to see God, focus on the heart center as if it were the center of our being.

Now, breathe there. Imagine that this is the source of kindness for the world. All kindness, all gentle wisdom springs forth from your heart. Radiate this healing energy out to heal the world.

Now, inhale into that. Then slowly exhale.

Now, focus on the core within the core of your heart, the source of your kindness, the place from where which it springs forth. Allow this kindness to radiate outward into the room. And now imagine that this source is the source of kindness for the entire world—the wellspring of kindness and compassion for the entire earth, the whole planet, for every creature. All kindness, all gentle wisdom springs forth from your heart. Radiate this healing energy out to heal the world.

And breathe . . .

This meditation can be revolutionary because if we focus on the darkness and hope the light comes in, our true focus is on the darkness, so that is what we continue to see. In other words, the mind is busy trying not to be busy. The human mind is so literal. But, if you focus on your heart, and seek the wellspring of kindness at its source, it could be said you've located the god/goddess within. You've become, in essence, the resting place, the temple of God. This practice will make you still and help you heal and quiet your mind. All of these powerful benefits occur as side effects because you have become the object you seek.

Step Three

Afterwards, be in no hurry to leave your meditation and reenter the material world. Do not rush away from your feelings. When you do finally go back out into the world, keep and cultivate this calmness so that when you meet others, they may become calm as a result of contact with you, instead of you becoming stressed from contact with them. In this simple way we can affect the world. In our own hearts we can reach out to heal the world and by doing so, heal ourselves.

EXERCISE --

A study revealed that the average attention span of an adult American is about twenty seconds. Fortunately, we can make a conscious effort to dramatically extend our attention span through practice. One of the meditation methods I teach is to ask you to visualize not just an object, but a person or thing in your life that you have immense gratitude for. That means you can focus on Jesus, or the Buddha, or you can focus on your grandmother or your two-month-old baby. Whatever it is, you choose. The point is to choose something that is immeasurably valuable to you on an emotional and spiritual level and then focus on it.

The symbol you choose is not ultimately the most important thing. The actual form is valuable only in its ability to direct your energies. What happens in your mind is what is important. If you think of your grandmother and she is the person you are most grateful for, your heart will swell, tears will come to your eyes, and you will feel filled with the highest of human emotions. The result is that now you are sitting with your heart open, filled with love, and your mind quiets.

So, to review: When meditating, rather than waiting for something to happen, understand that *you* are what is going to happen. You are the guest that's coming into the house. Don't wait for the guest; you are the guest.

--- •

Your Nervous System and the Beginning of Harmony

Why are we so stressed out? In the late-nineteenth and early-twentieth centuries, several yoga and Sufi masters traveled to the Western world, and each one commented on how due to industry, commerce, and machines, the Western mind was overwrought with stress. And this was even before the use of electricity was common, before the advent of telephones, automobiles, airplanes, and radio, and before the existence of television, computers, e-mails, and PDAs. What we think of as normal in this context is not even close to healthy. Our nervous system is not wired for this. Birds are not wired to see glass windows, deer are not wired to run across highways with cars zooming in straight lines at 70 miles per hour, and humans are not meant to stare all day at a flat illuminated surface with coffee triggering a fight-or-flight response in their body. Although we are able to adapt and do so, it would be false to say it is an optimum environment for our nervous system and physical well-being.

The nervous system comprises the brain, spinal cord, and nerves, and is a network that sends signals from one part of the body to another, coordinating our actions. Some of these actions are conscious, while others are subconscious.

A simple way to classify the nervous system is by dividing it into two parts:

1) The *somatic nervous system* is responsible for coordinating conscious or voluntary body movements, such as walking, speaking, and similar learned functions.

2) The *autonomic nervous system* is responsible for coordinating and harmonizing involuntary functions, such as the activity of the heart, the digestive system, and breathing. The autonomic nervous system can also be divided into two subsystems: the sympathetic nervous system, and the parasympathetic nervous system.

   a. The *sympathetic nervous system* responds to stress by speeding up the heart rate, constricting blood vessels, decreasing digestive activity, raising blood pressure, and preparing the body to fight or run (the fight-or-flight response). When it triggers the fight-or-flight response, it floods the body with hormones, particularly adrenaline. The fight-or-flight response can be useful in life-threatening or emergency situations. Even though we don't often encounter emergencies that require sudden and extreme physical effort in contemporary society, the body still creates fight-or-flight responses to emergencies.

   This means that we sometimes find our stress response activated in situations where physical action is unnecessary and/or inappropriate. For example, the fight response is associated with the emotion of anger, so it commonly manifests as hostile, argumentative behavior, while the flight response may manifest as social withdrawal and as addictions, including substance abuse, gambling, and chronic television viewing. Prolonged stress can also result in chronic suppression of the immune system. This can cause one to frequently contract colds or the flu, or, after long-term suppression, become unable to fight more-dangerous diseases. Also, if the sympathetic system is out of whack, the digestive system is also out of whack.

   b. The *parasympathetic nervous system*, or the "rest-and-digest" system, is concerned with nourishing, healing, and regeneration of the body, and counteracts the stress response by slowing the heart rate, increasing digestive and gland activity, and relaxing the muscles. The parasympathetic nervous system is activated by rest, relaxation, and positive thoughts. Studies have stated that moving yourself into the parasympathetic state, and staying there for as much time as possible, is essential for balanced living and for both physical and emotional healing.

The sympathetic and parasympathetic systems are antagonistic, and it is important to note that either one or the other is activated almost all of the time. The sympathetic system, however, instinctively takes precedence, because it is concerned with one's survival. It is easily triggered, for as soon as you think fearful or angry thoughts, or become too physically active, the body shifts into a sympathetic stance. So, in our modern world with its modern problems and stress, we must constantly seek to promote balance and healing by keeping the sympathetic system turned off as much as possible. This allows the maximum healing to occur. Simple ways to do this are to get seven to ten hours of sleep each night, take rests during the day, and replace negative thoughts with positive ones.

But we can do much more than this. It is possible to *consciously* still the mind and harmonize the nervous system. We can do this by utilizing our breathing practices, breath-initiated movement, and yoga postures, and, of course, meditation; in short, by following the Three Pillars of Transformation. This is why people who practice yoga, Qi Gong, and other internal practices are known for having vital health and a high level of energy yet a relaxed countenance, rather than a hyper or restless demeanor. This is because these practitioners are perhaps the only segment of society that consciously and regularly harmonizes their nervous systems.

We must remember that contemporary society as a whole exists in a state of unhealthy levels of stress and expectations, and although this has become what we call "normal," it could perhaps more accurately be called insane. It is our choice to acquiesce to this unhealthy way of stressful living, or to learn to consciously change our state to a harmonious one, regardless of the circumstances.

EXERCISE --

Five Things to Help You Relax in Two Weeks

> These techniques are to be done in tandem, and results should begin in two weeks or less. But this is more than a two-week experiment; these are new habits to aid you in staying relaxed as a new way of life. Becoming more relaxed will not disempower you or cause you to be less mentally sharp; conversely, living in a more-relaxed state will empower you, and help you to not only focus, but to also know what is important to focus on.

1) Listen or read the news once a week—no more. You will notice a difference in your nervous system in just a few days, and you may be surprised at what an addiction the news can be. From my own observation of myself and others, I believe that one of the most insidious sources of anxiety and stress is watching or reading the news every day. It is 99 percent negative, and when you really step back, you already know what the news is going to be the next time you see it. Since it's going to be essentially the same every day, why do we religiously bombard ourselves with such dark images of crisis? Only the names and locations change.

After drinking a triple latte and then heading out onto the freeway and listening to depressing news each and every day, it's no wonder so many people are on anti-ulcer drugs and antianxiety medication. Does this mean we should go into denial and ignore the problems? Absolutely not. Take action and do what you can to help. But during the rest of the week, do not obsess about the negative. If anything really momentous happens, you will hear about it; everyone will be talking about it, and then you can consult the media if you choose. This way, you can stay informed but not in a constant state of anxiety. The news plays up fear and conflict. Is that what you want to reinforce each day upon rising? Or the last thing you want to put in your imagination before sleeping? One of the most important contributions we can make to a troubled world is to give it more love, hope, and joy.

2) Read inspiring, life-affirming books before going to sleep at night—books by or about the greatest souls in history. Whether it is the Bible, the Upanishads, the Torah, the Koran, great philosophers, or inspiring poetry—to go to sleep with hope and inspiration will improve the quality of your sleep and dreams.

3) Watch no violent or disturbing images on TV or at the movies. No explanation is necessary.

4) Get to sleep by 10 PM. According to traditional Chinese medicine (those who practice acupuncture), the period of time between 10 PM and 3 AM is the most vital for the body to replenish and repair itself.

5) Give up caffeine gradually. Sorry, but it is important. You need to stop triggering the fight-or-flight response and somehow expect new results. Do so in steps, not cold turkey. Drink it only in the morning. Drink half a cup of coffee or half a latte and then pour out the rest. Switch to green or white tea with only water, no milk or soy milk. Then, if you can, gradually eliminate the tea as well. What will amaze you is that you will find you have more energy, not less.

FIVE

The Second Pillar—The Emotions

In ancient symbology, water is commonly used to symbolize both the emotions and also the Spirit, or Soul. Regarding the latter, rituals such as baptism signify the immersion of our Spirit into God's, whereas in the former, watery tears emerge from our eyes when emotions such as love, joy, and grief overflow. Alcoholic beverages are called "spirits," as they are known for evoking our emotions.

Your individual Spirit is the very foundation of your emotions, and it is the edifying or debasement of your Spirit that is at the root of your emotional state at any given time. Your emotions are the horses that draw the carriage forth. They power or disempower your decisions, taking them into action, or quelling them. Even your spiritual journey can be propelled or crushed by your emotions, so they must be trained and nourished, educated to follow your highest impulses while retaining their great ocean-like power.

Example: Your anger may cause you to act inappropriately and hurt someone close to you. Later, when you have calmed down, your hurtful actions cause you deep shame, and your very Spirit shrinks. But then listening to the impulse of your Spirit, you transform your shame into a quest for reconciliation and you ask for forgiveness. Your understanding transforms your arrogance to true humility. You are forgiven, and your heart bursts with gratitude. Your Spirit blossoms.

Your anger debased you, and then through humility, your desire for reconciliation lifted your Spirit up again. This is how emotional work is a form of important spiritual work.

What does it mean to train the emotions? It means to enhance your life at the very source of your actions, and to transform habitual negative emotions that damage you into higher emotions that elevate you. In this chapter you will explore the debilitating forces of anger, depression, and reactionary behavior, and learn about the powerful tools you already possess to bring yourself back into balance and beyond.

The undisciplined spirit does not act; it reacts. The undisciplined spirit succumbs to the emotions of others around it. Picture yourself going to a movie: If it is a comedy, you will laugh; if it is a tragedy, you will cry; if it is a thriller, you will become anxious. In all cases you are *reacting* to external stimulus. But you are the same outside the movie theater. If someone is angry toward you, you will become angry; if someone close to you is sad, you become sad. Your mind will also react to discomfort or pleasure in an automatic fashion. In this way you are like pinball machine: The ball hits a button and the button lights up and a lever is triggered.

Your happiness or unhappiness is actually a result of choices you make; often, you are not even aware that you are making them because they are triggered by external things. Once conscious and aware of this phenomenon, you can learn to see in a new way and also understand that you have the power to shift your state of mind, or state of being.

I was once stuck in an airport in one of those exceptionally inconvenient flight-delay stories. Just as I became somewhat agitated at the level of absurdity that was being displayed by the airline's policies, something happened: Many of the other passengers around me became far more agitated than I was, even furious. I saw grown men and women reduced to the behavior of pouting, snippy teenagers. One man threw a tantrum. The behavior all around me was shameful. Seeing this calmed me right down. I was determined not to become reactive like so many around me. It really hit home at that moment that we could be stuck in this airport and be angry, or we could be stuck in this airport and be happy. Either way, we were going to be stuck, and there was nothing we could do about it. I remembered that happiness is a choice, so, I chose to be happy. I sat down and began to read a book, and soon felt quite content.

It is a choice. It really is just a matter of getting a handle on our emotions within a situation, remembering that while circumstances are often beyond our control, our emotions are our own. The practice of choosing your state of mind is the beginning of happiness.

Depression

**Everything is going to be okay in the end—if it's not okay,
it's not the end.**
—Anonymous

Sadly, there are a staggering number of people who exist in a state of slow-burning misery, or they live a nihilistic life of anger-drenched grief, which the modern world calls depression. It has exploded like a plague, infecting millions each year, and perhaps indicates a social ailment that is underreported and understudied, and patients who are overly medicated. Depression is an evolving term in Western society.

In my opinion, depression can be divided into two major categories:

1) Clinical depression, which can be caused by a chemical imbalance, extreme trauma, or prolonged grief.
2) Dejection, gloomy sadness, lowness of spirit, withdrawal.

The following section deals with the second group. Because of the epidemic of emotional depression, the pharmaceutical industry is now one of the most profitable in America. To label depression as a disorder that should be medicated is making a lot of people in this industry very wealthy. You can now obtain these new medications from your family doctor without any kind of therapy or testing, and without agreeing to go to counseling or to commit to self-study of any kind. Put simply, doctors are now medicating unhappiness.

About 6 percent of American citizens were prescribed an antidepressant in 1996—13 million people—which then rose to more than 10 percent, or 27 million people, by 2005. Some believe that this figure has since doubled. It is indisputable that for many people, taking antidepressants has prevented them from committing suicide; for others, taking these drugs allowed them to climb out of a blackness that seemed inescapable, like someone in a pitch-black auditorium fumbling in the darkness for a way out. We can be truly thankful that we live in a time when these medications are available. But I also believe that the vast majority of people taking these new drugs belong to the second category; they have chosen to live, or rather exist, by using antidepressants as a coping technology rather than a healing technology. The first, coping, implies stasis, while healing implies positive transformation.

If you tell your doctor that you are depressed and would like medication for it, using different words, you are saying, "I am chronically unhappy and I don't know what to do." This is an important first step in changing—recognizing that you are acutely or habitually depressed. This is good, because it means you are turning your face toward *what is*, toward the truth. But could it be that the depression itself isn't the problem; rather, that it's the problem that is causing the depression? I propose that for a great many people, depression is a healthy symptom, just as other types of pain are symptoms. If you accidentally put your hand on a hot stove and you shout in anguish, pain is the body's signal to get your hand off the burner, and prescribing pain medication would be one way of dealing with it. Similarly, depression can be a symptom that is telling you that you need to make some changes in your life. Perhaps you can consider another way of dealing with your depression that is safer and more effective. Sometimes we need to heal our energetic heart center, not cover healthy symptoms with medication.

I once worked with a yoga student—I'll call her Catherine—who was fairly successful on the material plane. One day she confided in me about her life. She said, "You know, I'm good at my work; I make enough money, and I live in a nice house in the hills. But I've realized that I don't like my work anymore. I haven't liked it for ten years. I keep doing it because I'm good at it and I get a decent amount of money for it and my family has grown accustomed to a certain lifestyle. We're not rich but we're pretty comfortable. These days, my marriage isn't going well anymore, either, and I find that I'm now depressed most of the time. My doctor wants to put me on medication. What do you think?" (Does this remind you of the ox story?)

I thought to myself, This is a terribly sad story with so much misunderstanding of priorities. I told Catherine that it sounded like perhaps she needed to consider making some changes. She answered that she was afraid to, and she felt she didn't have the courage to make radical changes in her life. I gently expressed my opinion: I didn't feel medication was the answer for her. I said, "From what you've described, you *should* be depressed. It's a natural and healthy response to the situation that you've just laid out to me. You just described that you've been living a life you no longer want to live—for several years. For God's sake, you need to make some changes. Ignoring the fact that your situation is ruining you emotionally and then taking drugs to deal with the emotions that are being ignored sounds like it will only exacerbate the situation and not heal it."

I suggested that perhaps Catherine might consider another way of dealing with her depression, including finding a new therapist, and taking a sabbatical (she was due for one) so that she might have the time and energy necessary to analyze her life, her feelings, and her marriage. She would have the time to practice her yoga—and especially her breathing techniques—every day. Doing so would open her up again to her inner life, and perhaps with the help of an effective therapist, the answers would be revealed.

For Catherine, taking medication for depression as a first course of action made as much sense as someone complaining of intense chest pains dealing with it by taking pain relievers and then going on with their stressful routine. Chest pain means a heart attack may be imminent. In my opinion, people like Catherine need to work on healing the energetic heart, not covering healthy symptoms with medication.

I have taught breath-centered practices to people who are depressed and have seen significant breakthroughs time and time again. A four-day-a-week yoga practice, with extra emphasis on breath-work, will nearly always ignite a shift in your perception of your life and give you the clarity and context you need for making new choices. Finding a talented therapist is also important, with an emphasis on mutual trust and respect.

G. I. Gurdjieff said the most powerful energy is that energy which has been transformed from negative into positive. To learn to consciously transform our outlook from depressed to inspired is one of the great achievements of a lifetime. It is in suffering we have the opportunity to learn how to transform our misery into joy, our despair into gratitude, and our cynicism into wisdom

Wisdom requires context. What limits your understanding of your life is the extremely narrow context through which you process the events and experiences. As you age and progress with your work in self-inquiry, your context will expand, and events that you previously defined as negative will often be seen with new eyes as ultimately positive. The toy you long ago felt was the ultimate treasure, you now feel nothing about. The car you coveted as a teenager now is simply an amusing memory. The lover you once believed you could not live without, you are now deeply grateful is not part of your life. As your context enlarges, so does your ability to understand life. This is why we constantly redefine meaning and fulfillment as we age. During difficult times, you need to recall the toy, the car, the indispensable relationship, and know that one day in the future, you may look at your present circumstances and simply smile.

Another indispensable step toward magnifying our vision and therefore our wisdom is to read of wisdom traditions from around the world. Studying sacred texts or writings of great souls helps to broaden our vision of mankind, the world, and God, and enables us to see the world less as a one-dimensional cardboard cutout, and more as a three-dimensional matrix.

Traveling to foreign lands and visiting cultures different from our own also illuminates life. We learn that life in our nation is not the only version of the human experience, and we also learn that there are certain aspects of these foreign cultures we enjoy or respect more than our own. We begin to see our culture at home as *a* culture, and not the culture. This cultivates tolerance and a life vision rooted in personal experience and not in fear.

If traveling to foreign lands is not possible, you might try visiting areas of your city (or another nearby city) that is very different from your own. Many cities have immigrant communities where you could swear you were instead in their home country. You may feel a little afraid of doing this at first, only to find later that you have as much or more in common with this new culture than you do with your own.

Anger

When you are mad at somebody, you're mad at everybody; at least you behave that way. For instance, if you honk your car horn in anger at one person, everyone around you hears it. Consciously or not, you punish everyone with your irritable mood; you are, to a certain degree, infecting everybody else.

> We are not punished for our anger; we are punished
> by our anger.
> —The Buddha

When we built Sacred Movement Yoga in Los Angeles, we had a challenge with noise from the busy four-lane street just outside. During rush hour, commuter traffic would get backed up, creating an unpleasant rumble. So, we replaced the windows with glass blocks, which let the light in and kept most of the noise out. The one noise that would still sometimes pierce through was that of honking horns.

One day near the end of my class, when everyone was resting in their final relaxation pose (*shavasana*), I was sitting in front of the class and observing everyone in their peaceful state. It was one of those classes where at the end, it just looked like everybody was in heaven. I was grateful to see everybody resting so peacefully. Then, in this great moment, somebody outside decided to lean on his or her horn as loudly as possible. (I don't know how they design horns, but you can always tell if somebody's really angry, can't you?)

When the horn honked I saw the entire class of nearly fifty students jump, for it startled everyone. I saw all fifty nervous systems startle and tense. Some students even opened their eyes and looked around before eventually trying to settle back down. Seeing this occur made me ponder, because it was really quite interesting.

Had I been able to, I would have walked outside and knocked on the car window of the driver who had honked his horn. I would have gestured for the driver to roll down his window, and I would have asked him, "Are you aware that you just honked your horn really loudly?" And he would have said, "Of course; I was honking at this so-and-so in front of me. The light's been green for two and a half seconds, and he's still sitting there."

And then I would have said, "But are you aware that when you honked your horn at that driver, you startled everyone in the cars all around you? And, in fact, there's a yoga center right there, with fifty people that all jumped up in the air when you honked your horn? And you know what else? We have two yoga rooms. In the other room there are thirty-five people; I'm quite sure they were startled as well. And you probably aren't aware of this, but next door to our yoga center, there's a bodywork center with a host of people relaxing on massage tables; I'm certain that they were disturbed as well. And if you just look around the block here, there are several restaurants and stores, and apartments above the stores—so I estimate that six or seven hundred people felt your horn blast."

When we honk our horn in anger at one person, everyone around us feels it equally. When we're mad at one person, we behave like we're mad at everybody.

Try talking to someone who has just been in a shouting match with somebody; full of adrenaline, they might turn and yell at you. It is common when someone tries to break up a fistfight that the peacemaker gets hit as well, because the person who's swinging just keeps on swinging. They don't care—they're mad at everybody at that point.

But you and I are like that too. If you have a really bad day at work and then you go home to your husband or wife, you probably share your frustrations. We call it venting. And at some point your husband or wife may look at you and say, "What are you yelling at me for? I didn't do it." And you yell back, "I know you didn't do it! And I'm not yelling!" Have you experienced this before? On both ends, probably. This is actually quite significant, because resentment is the accumulation of anger carried over time, and as we carry this little vial of resentment everywhere we go, chances are we're sharing it with everybody, especially our immediate family.

Remember: We can affect our relationships positively, or infect them negatively. Negative emotions can spread though a family or community like an infectious disease. But healing spreads through a community too.

Justifiable Hostility

Learn not to define yourself by what you are against;
instead, define yourself by expressing with your actions
and your words what you are for. It is easy to criticize,
but this has little value, for it is usually not wanted, and
therefore not listened to. It is of more benefit to praise that
which is praiseworthy, to speak of the greatness of things.
There are plenty of others to do the criticizing.

Most of us can be kind to others when they are being kind to us, but when someone insults us, then we often lose all sympathy and react with equal or greater unkindness as we challenge the offender to improve their behavior. But of course, they do not hear our intent because we are speaking in a tone of anger and self-righteousness, so they lash out again and the situation is now twice as bad as it was. Sound familiar?

The most destructive part is that we feel justified to be disrespectful because "They were unkind first." (Don't we teach our children that "Two wrongs don't make a right?") So, in our self-righteousness we place ourselves and others into a little hell-realm. Our entire body feels restless and ill, our expression is bitter, our mood dark and irritable, and we feel quite sanctimonious about it all. We can stew about it for hours, days, months, and even decades, and we will even act rudely to innocent people, sometimes those we love the most. So, hostility is an enemy of the seeker of peace, especially justifiable hostility, because that is when we act in a hostile manner and instead of feeling shame, we feel righteous in doing so.

Tolerance for the Angry

It can be sad to witness a beautiful being shrink in fear at the prospect of healing their emotions, and of embodying what they have said they want most. It is easy to lose patience with them and even to condemn them as hypocrites. Perhaps you tell them, "You say you are dedicated to peace, but every week I see you lose your temper and yell at somebody—including me." But it is not your place to condemn anyone for not being ready to change. It is easy for you to see what needs to be done, but life-changing for them to do. Besides, it may not be their time to transform yet, or maybe there's even a hidden reason for their frozen state. Either way, you are not to judge. Tolerance is at the core of this practice. If someone is not willing to heal today, you must answer with a willingness to wait for him or her forever. That being said, you may need to remove yourself from contact with him or her while you are waiting in order to protect yourself, while in your mind you patiently trust that change will come, and one day in the future you will meet again as friends. Your degree of intolerance for another's anger or fear is an indicator of your own intolerance.

Spiritual transformation is mysterious, and we must always remember this so that we do not impose timetables on others. I have observed students who appear to not grow or change for years. Week after week Bob came to class and didn't seem to learn anything. If I showed you a video of his tenth time practicing yoga and compared it with his three-hundredth time, you wouldn't see any difference. Bob appeared to not learn anything no matter what I said to him or how much special direction I gave him. People around him soared forth, blooming like a field of flowers. Bob stayed the same. And then suddenly, one day, Bob seemed to have a major epiphany; I saw a radical transformation occur within him that spun his practice and his life in a radically new direction. It was as if he had unconsciously been building up enough energy over the span of three years to make the change. I have seen this happen many times.

When someone is put into your life, in your face, who repulses you by their actions, perhaps they are there as an example, to teach you what *not* to do. Without these people you would never really learn about anger, irritability, patience, compassion, and forgiveness. For example, when someone is behaving rudely to you, it is easy to forget in an instant everything you have ever learned on your spiritual path. To keep centered can be very challenging. I have found that an effective way to keep centered is to look at them as if they were physiologically impaired. If they were physically impaired you know you would treat them compassionately; it is the same way with the physiologically impaired. You must have great compassion for their impairment and hope that their practice heals them. The critical, condemning mind gives way to the forgiving heart.

Have great patience and set boundaries—not electric fences, but kind, firm boundaries. In addition, we should try to choose close friends and confidants who are kind and considerate, moral and accountable, for they have the most direct influence over us and we over them.

Healing Your Own Anger Issues

1) First, consider eliminating caffeine from your diet; this culprit is notorious for eliciting reactionary behavior. If you are not sure whether it changes your behavior, ask someone close to you; he or she will tell you.

2) If you feel that you tend to be competitive or aggressive by nature, I recommend that you avoid yoga classes that approach "attaining" postures as the main focus. Instead, seek out classes that are noncompetitive and more oriented toward healing. Release your addiction to "power" and seek out breath and alignment. You will discover a new kind of power that will astonish you.

3) Remember to set your intention at the beginning of your practice every day. An intention is a purpose; define it for yourself. This is easy to do and has extraordinarily positive consequences. If you want to be more loving to your children, what could you say to yourself before the practice? Perhaps something like "I breathe for my children. I awaken the love within me." Keep hold of your intention in your heart as you practice, and breathe into your heart so your highest ideal pervades the body with every breath. Keep your breathing deep but not harsh. The jaw and tongue should remain relaxed.

4) The most powerful way to rid your body of intolerance and anger is the practice of forgiveness. This may be your root issue. (See section on forgiveness, page 72.)

--- •

Overreacting

One of the most common and destructive behaviors is overreacting, especially, ironically, with your loved ones. Here's an example:

Sarah and John

Sarah does something benign but her husband John takes offense. Unbeknownst to Sarah, John's feelings are hurt, and he points out the offending act with a sharp tone. Sarah, not understanding why John is suddenly speaking to her with a sharp tone, feels attacked, and defends herself by launching a counterattack. Now we have an argument, and neither John nor Sarah really understand what is going on other than the fact that they both feel innocent of any wrongdoing and unjustly attacked. After a period of heated words, a calmer discussion sorts it all out, and after a few days life goes back to normal. Sound familiar?

EXERCISE --

When someone you care about appears to offend you, stop. Think: I know it is possible I am misinterpreting what just happened. Do I really believe he/she suddenly doesn't love me? No. I know he/she loves me deeply and means no harm.

Next: As calmly as possible, say something like this to your partner: "I think I am misunderstanding what you mean; would you say it again in a different way?"

If you still feel like the other person is attacking, then try: "I know you don't mean it this way, but you are speaking in a way that is a little intense. Maybe you don't realize it. If you wouldn't mind, let's take a few moments and then you can talk about it. I do want to talk, but after a few minutes."

Usually arguments are all about feeling hurt by the tone of what was said more than *what* was said. This is why you often don't remember what you fought about a few days later, because it wasn't so much about the actual words but how you emotionally reacted to the tone of voice and body language of the other person. So, when angry or hurt, avoid going over the details. Address only the miscommunication and forgive the situation. You can then discuss the original topic when you both are calm.

Peace is not only the absence of war, but also a way of seeing the world, and the choices we make are how we express and manifest that vision of the world.

--- •

Forgiveness

The choice is simple: to forgive or to resent. Forgiveness brings peace; resentment fosters pain within and eventually expresses itself as harmful behavior and health issues. It is simply a choice—the choice of your life.

No matter how many vinyasas we do, no matter how much wheatgrass juice we drink, no matter how many kirtans we attend, we will not have a happy life if we are carrying resentment and hatred inside us. For the body to heal, oftentimes what is most vital is to heal the broken heart or spirit. Failure to forgive affects our stress level, our power to heal the body, our discernment, and all of our relationships. There are other infectious diseases as tragic as AIDS or smallpox. Anger is infectious, and hatred is infectious, and if we invest emotionally in the cycle of vengeance instead of forgiveness, then we are doomed, and our children are doomed as we pass along our negative emotions to our families.

The antidote for these infections is forgiveness—perhaps the most powerful tool we have for healing ourselves—for to forgive another heals oneself, just as anger toward another poisons oneself.

FORGIVE (v): 1. to renounce anger or resentment against; 2. to give up desire or power to punish.

Many of us are unhappy in life, and no matter how much we exercise, entertain ourselves, or practice yoga, we still go to bed unhappy and sleep poorly, or wake up in the middle of the night, anxious and despairing. Eventually you may discover that you need to forgive someone before you can sleep at night. Medication may appear to solve the problem but it doesn't; even meditating may not solve the problem because you might be sitting on a volcano. So, until you forgive those who have harmed you, or who you perceive have harmed you, you will not have a happy life. And you will not be as good of a parent, spouse, friend, or leader as you could be.

In addition to causing your own suffering, holding anger affects and infects all of your relationships. The happier you become, the more positively you will affect those around you. The more resentment you hold, the more negatively you will affect others. If you do not learn to forgive others, you will be perpetually filled with resentment, and this resentment will harm you, and could eventually, in essence, poison you to death. This manifests as many kinds of illnesses, like heart disease, and can also lead to dangerous addictions that lead to ill health and a shortened life span. For example, one large study found that among 12,986 middle-aged men and women, those who rated high in traits such as anger but had normal blood pressure were more prone to coronary artery disease (CAD) or heart attack. In fact, the angriest people faced roughly twice the risk of CAD and almost three times the risk of heart attack compared to subjects with the lowest levels of anger.

As long as we are stuck in seething resentment, we are in a self-imposed prison, even a hell-realm. I myself have spent time in that prison. It was as if I had swallowed a red-hot coal, and that coal sat burning in my gut—but I refused to spit it up, so the coal just kept burning. To release myself from this prison-hell, I had no choice but to forgive.

Be clear that to forgive does not mean to go into denial, condone, or forget. To forgive also does not mean to sublimate or repress your anger. When the anger is new it should be expressed—appropriately. In some cases therapy may be invaluable, particularly with traumatic cases. But once the anger has been acknowledged, expressed, and processed, then we begin the process of forgiveness.

What Isn't Forgiveness?

Forgiveness does not mean you forget. If you walk down a path and are bitten by a snake, you should forgive that snake, but wisdom dictates that you don't forget where the snake lives, and therefore, you choose to walk down a different path.

Forgiveness does not mean denial. It does not mean that you pretend no wrong was committed.

Forgiveness does not mean you have no boundaries. It is difficult to speak about love and boundaries separately, for boundaries are an intelligent expression of love. Many believe, mistakenly, that love or true friendship knows no boundaries, but from my experience, you must be willing at times to say no as an expression of love. Just like with a toddler: If a two-year-old picks up a sharp knife or matches, you must say "no" to her and take the dangerous objects away. To allow a two-year-old to play with a sharp knife or matches isn't loving behavior—it is neglect. Similarly, if an adult is causing harm to you, you must be willing to say "no" to that person, and at times even exclude him from your daily life. Your circle of love must include yourself, and you must avoid letting others mistreat you. You can do this by speaking out, kindly but firmly when necessary. This doesn't mean you should meet anger with anger; it means you must communicate truth with the kindness and strength you feel is appropriate. But again, sometimes the wise and loving thing to do is to avoid someone's company altogether and remove them from your daily life.

Most important, forgiveness does not mean that you condone or approve of the harmful action committed. The belief that forgiveness means that you now condone the harmful behavior is why, I believe, so many of us will not forgive. There are so many of us who could tell stories of unbelievable tragedy—wrongs committed against us, or against our loved ones; wrongs that we will never approve or condone, nor should we.

But there is a vast difference between forgiving and condoning. To quote a friend who spoke of his own struggle to forgive his father, who had abused him:

When I think of my father and the abuses he committed, I ardently reject his shameful behavior and the suffering he caused with all my soul. And had I been old enough to even know that his actions weren't my fault, I would have tried to stop him. Now, in my life and through my work, I try to educate others not to think or act in such a way as he. But I still forgive him. The only other choice—to resent and hate him—would torture me. Destroy me. This means his long arm of cruelty would reach my heart and crush it until I become a vessel of wrath, more like him than not.

What Is Forgiveness?

Forgiveness means: *I let it go. I let the pain and anger and infectious poison of resentment leave my body. I pull the thorn from my heart. I spit out the red-hot coal I have swallowed. I release it.*

There are many who say, "But some things are unforgivable!" If this is true, then you have condemned yourself to a lifetime of suffering, reliving the past painful event over and over. It is said that when someone causes great harm to you, you are the victim. But each time you replay the crime in your mind, you are harming yourself. You are controlled by the past. You are still controlled by the person who harmed you. It is like you are in a prison of your own making, and the person who harmed you is your jailer.

> **To understand everything is to forgive everything.**
> **—The Buddha**

> **Forgive them, for they know not what they do . . .**
> **—Jesus of Nazareth**

If one considers the life of the Mahatma Gandhi, one might say that he had plenty to be angry about—more than many of us. He lived in a country that was colonized by a foreign empire known for its flagrant exploitation of people and resources, resulting in massive poverty, human rights abuses, and corruption in India. Hundreds of Gandhi's countrymen and -women were gunned down, and thousands were brutally beaten during peaceful protests, while Gandhi himself was imprisoned several times—once for as long as two years. His beloved wife died after eighteen months of imprisonment.

According to the doctrine of "But some things are unforgivable," one could certainly argue that Gandhi had plenty of reasons to be angry and even to hate. But that wasn't the case. He was a peaceful and kind person—in fact, he was renowned for his kind demeanor. Was he in denial? On the contrary; he dedicated most of his life to restoring his people and country to independence. He was the ultimate activist. But he seemed to forgive the perpetrators as he struggled against them, and that is why he is now an archetype of a peaceful and kind human being. Gandhi was an activist for change, *and* he was a peaceful and happy person.

When we grant mercy to others, we set an example of mercy. When we grant mercy to others, we grant mercy to ourselves. When we forgive another, releasing them from our negative tempest, we release ourselves from a kind of slavery to the past.

I once led a guided meditation at the end of a class where I intuitively felt called to speak about forgiveness. I said simply this: "Choose someone in your life that you have been harboring resentment toward, someone you have had a very difficult time forgiving, and try to practice forgiveness tonight. Knowing that as you let go and forgive them, as you soften your heart toward them, you are also softening your heart toward the world and toward yourself. Knowing that when you do not forgive someone, there is part of you that won't forgive yourself for something. By healing this wound between you and the other person— even if you don't say it to them out loud—by doing this, you are truly healing part of yourself."

About a month later a student who was in that class came up to me and said that she had really gotten angry with me for saying that, because she focused on someone in her life who had abused her. But when she finally did decide to forgive that person, it actually led her to make a phone call after years of silence. She talked out this relationship and brought it to a new level; there was forgiveness and even reconciliation that came out of this process. The reluctance to ask for forgiveness or to offer forgiveness is commonplace, but when one witnesses a person forgiving another, it is so beautiful that one cannot be unmoved.

This aforementioned event serves to eternally remind me that we should all trust our intuition. Sometimes we feel an internal calling just to say a few simple words. These simple words may inevitably resound with someone and spark an act of love, kindness, or forgiveness. So, in this way, words spoken from the heart in their moment of conception can help to better the world. If you say something that resounds in another human being and they turn to someone they have had a dispute with and they reconcile that dispute, then they are both healed a little, and they are both likely to heal another wound because of the success of that reconciliation. This can start a domino effect of healing, and as you know, anything that "dominos" through human beings does so exponentially.

This is an example of the power of love, and how words spoken from your heart can carry that message of love. The key, of course, is having the courage to speak from your heart. When you speak from your heart it makes you very vulnerable, but vulnerability is what we are asking for from others, so we have to be able to set an example.

Self-forgiveness

It is virtually impossible to live this life without making errors. If you are born, live, and die in this world without making any big mistakes, a new religion will spring up around you, because that is how often it occurs. Almost never.

Do you hold yourself up to impossible standards? Where did that come from—your parents? And if so, have they met their own impossible standards? And are they happy? Because this is an important litmus test to assess whether or not their system works.

Who else are you comparing yourself to? Study more closely the lives of your heroes. We tend to mythologize our heroes, believing them to be infallible. Study their lives more carefully and you will see that they also made errors; they, too, experienced shame, guilt, and regret.

And finally, don't presume to know the long-term outcome of your errors, because you don't really know. Sometimes our worst mistakes become blessings to others years later.

I want to share a true story that might illustrate this. Imagine Germany in the late 1800s. Like most of Europe at that time, it was a royalist empire ruled by hierarchies. It was a place where the few ruled the many through a distinct and rigid class system, where human rights, wages, and laws differed depending on which class you belonged to. The wealthy all had house servants from the lower classes, and this story is about a particular good-hearted young German woman from humble origins, named Clara.

Clara went to work as a housemaid in the home of a wealthy merchant. The merchant had a son who became very interested in their lovely young servant, and they began an affair. We do not know whether her relationship with the merchant's son was consensual or not, because in those days, masters of the house saw it as their right to engage in sexual activity with their female servants, and it was not an issue protected by the laws we know today. But there was reason to believe that they felt strongly about each other. Eventually Clara found herself pregnant.

When the father learned of their relationship and Clara's pregnancy, it was a scandal, threatening to tarnish the family name, and the son was banished to America. As for Clara, she was given a little money and dismissed from her position. In those days this was a misfortune that would change the course of Clara's life. For now she was an unmarried woman, with child, and without prospects. She faced disgrace, gossip, and a disreputable name. Her chances of marrying were now virtually gone, and with an infant to take care of, it would be extremely difficult for her to earn a living.

Let us step back and imagine what Clara was thinking and feeling. She was angry, despondent, and shamed. Worst of all, she blamed herself. She easily could have felt that she had destroyed her life and it was all her fault. Now, what was she going to do with a child? How could she have been so stupid? She was wracked with guilt. To Clara, this was the biggest mistake of her life, and it was unforgivable. From her young perspective, she probably saw no good coming from this, and that would be an understandable point of view. We don't know a lot about how she pulled things together, but somehow she did. Clara raised her son and he became a man she could be proud of.

I, for one, am grateful that Clara kept and raised her child, for that child was my grandfather, and Clara was my great-grandmother. I wish I could thank her because I know her journey wasn't easy. I am also sure that because she saw her son grow to become a good-hearted person just as she was, she understood that ultimately he was not a mistake, but her greatest treasure.

When we are young and have almost no wisdom, we all make poor choices, and, sometimes, terrible ones. Most of the time we are lucky and there are no consequences—or, at least, no lasting ones. And then sometimes we are not so lucky. When I was twenty-one years old, I was driving home alone after an exhausting and stressful day. I was driving on one of the most treacherous freeways in Northern California, known for its winding turns and head-on collisions. I fell sound asleep at the wheel.

The mistake? I knew I was drowsy but believed I could stay awake; I should have pulled over and slept for a while. The consequence? I awoke as my car plowed through a grassy field at fifty miles an hour. No one was harmed, apart from the grass. Not even my car was damaged. That night I was lucky. My car swerved to the right and safely into the field. It could have just as easily swerved to the left and killed a family in an oncoming car. The error was the same regardless of the consequences. Sometimes our destiny leads us out of harm's way, and sometimes it leads us right into it. You may blame yourself for causing great harm, and even though you have made amends, you still carry the weight of guilt on your heart, unable to forgive yourself.

Remember: Forgiveness cannot repair the past, but it *can* repair your heart and mind, and it can prepare you to make the best choices now. If you have not left this world yet, then there is more for you to do. Make amends, forgive yourself, learn from your mistakes, and then begin again.

You may have made your error (or errors) because, for a time or a moment, you misunderstood the purpose of life on Earth. But in this life you can be reborn several times. Many saints and spiritual teachers began as people who misunderstood the purpose of this life and who caused others harm, but then they rose again from their tragedies, or confusion, or anger, and began a completely new life. Saint Paul was a classic example of this. Prior to his conversion to Christianity, Paul (then named Saul) violently persecuted the church of God. He was a powerful man who intentionally caused great harm to others. "Saul began to destroy the church. Going from house to house, he dragged off men and women and put them in prison" (Acts 8:3). After putting these people in prison, Saul learned about their Christian friends in Damascus by somehow getting letters from the prisoners.

"I persecuted the followers of this Way to their death, arresting both men and women and throwing them into prison, as also the high priest and all the Council can testify. I even obtained letters from them to their brothers in Damascus, and went there to bring these people as prisoners to Jerusalem to be punished" (Acts 22:4–5).

Saul was on a zealous mission. It was not an accident, such as drinking too much one night, or forgetting to take your birth control pills. Saul did these acts with eyes wide open and with pride. I think it is safe to say that before his conversion, Saul did not understand the heart of this world, of God, or of his own soul. But Saul began again after his conversion; he was forgiven and he forgave himself, and he went on to live an exemplary life. Today he is called Saint Paul the Apostle and his words are studied as a major part of the New Testament.

As a young man, Francis of Assisi went to war as a soldier, before his gradual awakening. Eventually he was transformed into the ultimate pacifist, Saint Francis of Assisi. But it did not happen for him all at once; first, he experienced years of confusion and distress.

Therefore, do not harbor resentment and guilt toward yourself; forgive yourself as well as everyone else. Do you think the world really needs you to be crippled with guilt? Learn from your errors. Make a pledge to change. Transform from a victim to an activist. Make amends, and, if appropriate, work to help those you have harmed. There are many people who need you, especially your spouse and your children. And they need you whole and happy. We all need you that way.

The practice of forgiving yourself and others is daily work. You will likely need to do it again, even after you think it is finished.

EXERCISE ---
Posture: Headstand. Headstand is a wonderful antidote for anger and calming the spirit. Practice it six days a week. To begin, be sure to learn under the guidance of an experienced teacher.

--- •

Remember: Forgiveness is daily work; you will likely need to do it again even after you think it is finished. You are replacing the daily practice of re-angering yourself with forgiveness.
Remember: Never assume that you know someone's intention. We are often incorrect in our assumptions. Forgive the person but not the action.
Remember: One does not need to have the other person present to forgive them.

Prayer: *Forgive him/her, for they know not what they do ... I release him/her—knowing their action was born from misunderstanding. Ultimately we are the same. We both have failed to love and to understand, and we both*

have good hearts. I know we will meet again, with a new
and clear knowledge and understanding, and we will
drop all enmity. We will understand this life, and we will
ultimately be friends.

The Opportunities of Catastrophes

Catastrophes, as challenging as they can be, can create new, unexpected opportunities. We can reinterpret a negative situation into a wake-up call for action. When tragedy strikes, find your footing and let the dust settle. Then, in a few days, take some time and try to see the event from different points of view. Often when things explode in your face, they also blow open new doors. And one of these new doors may just be the answer to your prayer. It was just delivered more powerfully and suddenly than you would have liked.

Sometimes when your life falls apart, it is because it's not held together with consciousness, but rather with illusion, and so it crumbles. What is left is actually a clearer vision of what is real and of value. Many people have found their life's path only after what they had formerly perceived as their life had crumbled to dust. In other words, it is the illusion of your life that crumbles, leaving reality in its place. For example, often when people lose their jobs and they perceive it as a tragedy, they are forced to reassess and begin again. And sometimes they find that the new path they've chosen is the career they were waiting for their entire life. In difficult times, we are revealed to ourselves.

Stay courageous. To have your courage stripped away by others is something you cannot afford to let happen. Money and property can be taken away by others, but your strength of spirit and human goodness is yours alone to keep or give away.

Gratitude, the Parent of all Virtues

Gratitude seems to be one of the few transformational practices that unites people beyond beliefs and words—beyond nation, race, and tribe. It is really this simple: When you have a heart full of gratitude, your behavior is positive and kind, and when your heart is full of negative emotions, it is because you have lost your gratitude. To focus on gratitude and not on what you perceive to have lost is ultimately your choice, and it is perhaps the most important choice for your happiness and the happiness of those around you.

Imagine this: You are on vacation, resting languidly on a hammock between two palm trees on a gorgeous island in the South Pacific. The weather is perfect. Everything is perfect, peaceful, relaxing, and nourishing to the soul. On one side of you is a cozy grass hut, and on the other side is calm turquoise water of unspeakable beauty. It is easy to imagine that in these ideal and natural circumstances you would feel absolutely wonderful. To feel a deep sense of gratitude for what you have would not be challenging here.

But now, imagine this: While you are resting here on your island paradise, you are thinking about your problems back home—the same ones you dwell on every day. Now, there you are in paradise, with a sour expression and hard breath, your mind churning as your jaw tightens, and your paradise transforms energetically to your own private hell-realm.

The moral of this story is that when we lose our gratitude, we lose everything. It doesn't matter where you are if you do not feel gratitude; you may as well be back at your office. When you are feeling negative, it doesn't matter if you are in paradise; and if you are feeling gratitude, it doesn't matter if you are in difficult circumstances. Remember: Gratitude is accessible at any time, in any place; it is a choice to feel it or not.

This is how it works: When a room is dark and you open a window, allowing the sun to fill the room with light, the darkness flees. So, the dark heart, suffering from resentment or sorrow, need only focus sincerely on an image that invokes profound gratitude. It is not enough to "think of gratitude;" one must also focus on a person or thing which invokes this moving emotion—the more specific, the better. Gratitude is always within our grasp.

This is what I call *finding your center of gratitude*. Imagine that you are having a private session with a spiritual teacher. You have practiced some postures and breathing, but the teacher has noticed that you seem to be in a negative state. In fact, you have had a very difficult day, and you are harboring anger and upset within you.

So, you are sitting on your meditation cushion with your eyes closed and the teacher says, "Try and feel love; focus on love in your heart. Can you feel that?"

Your immediate response is, "No, not today. I feel no love."

So, the teacher changes her suggestion: "Then try and feel compassion for humanity. Focus on compassion."

You try for a moment, and then you admit, "No, I can't feel it. Not today. I am too angry."

The teacher then suggests, "Then perhaps what you need to do is to focus on forgiveness. Focus on forgiving the person or persons you are angry with. Can you do this?"

You just shake your head slowly. "Especially not forgiveness. I'm sorry, I am just being honest."

The teacher pauses, and then gently asks, "Then can you think of one person, or even one thing in the whole world, that you feel grateful for? Just one?"

You pause for a moment. Then you see the face of someone you love very much, someone who has only been good to you, someone who has been there for you in the worst of times. You realize that even in your current angry state, the image of this beloved person comes to mind. You are reluctant to allow it, but you slowly nod your head. "Yes, I am thinking of someone now."

The teacher continues: "Imagine this person sitting before you, smiling at you. Allow yourself to feel the gratitude you have for this person, and radiate this gratitude toward them. Wordlessly radiate the depths of your gratitude so he or she knows how you feel. Imagine them receiving it—and tears coming to their eyes."

From imagining this, your chest nearly bursts with gratitude, and when this happens, your heart fills with love and respect for your beloved friend. You sit now, full of love and humility instead of anger. The anger was dissolved and replaced by a higher emotion.

This is a technique I use with my students nearly every day. It is a very simple way of profoundly altering our emotional state from upset to deep gratitude in a matter of minutes. This exercise is available to you twenty-four hours a day, for the rest of your life, and it is one of the most powerful tools you own. Will you choose to use it?

You need only find the face of a person (or being) who is indispensable to your joy—whether it is the eyes of your child or your image of God—for this practice to transform your state from a living hell to one of living fulfillment and inner peace. When a dark heart fills with gratitude, love and humility instantaneously follow, and the heart becomes illuminated. This is why it is almost impossible for you to feel anger and gratitude at the same time.

Within your gratitude is one of your greatest powers, for only when you find gratitude do you begin to be liberated. Gratitude humbles you, and that humility enables you to forgive. Forgiveness gives birth to sympathy and love itself, and in love we are Liberated. Whether we call it Christ-consciousness, Buddha-consciousness, or the vision of Allah, let us remember our most profound gratitude, and forgive those who have forgotten theirs.

EXERCISE --
Practice *finding your center of gratitude* (explained above) daily, remembering that the human heart cannot hold gratitude and negative emotions at the same time. From gratitude, joy and all other virtues are born.

-- •

The Heart Center

We own nothing in this world. Everything we own is contained in our heart center, so spirituality is ultimately a mystical experience and not an academic one. It is where we keep all of our treasures, the container of what is truly our own. Everything outside the heart center is not ours. It passes. It's temporary. Everything in the heart center is real. The love we have for others, the love we feel from others, all resides in the heart center. It is the place where we sometimes experience the greatest pain, but it is also the fountain from which unconditional love flows—where joy, gratitude, forgiveness, and compassion are born.

The heart center is not a physical organ that beats in our chest; it is the temple of our highest emotions and even our highest Self. It is experienced primarily in the chest region, and this is why the chest is the most difficult area of the body to open, because it is the home of our emotions and our memories. All spiritual healing involves the heart center. It is where we truly live and will return to in the end.

The ancient Egyptians believed that the heart was the center of intelligence and emotion. They also thought so little of the brain that during mummification, they removed the brain from the body and discarded it.

Kindness is one of the expressions of the heart center; it is love in action. Kindness says to others, "You are also important; my concern is not just for my own well-being, but for yours also." This isn't easy for our ego-mind, for to accept that others are equally important feels like death to the ego. But kindness has immense power. No kindness is small. Think back to when you were a child or a teenager, and recall a simple act of kindness that someone did for you. Now, as you relive this beautiful moment in your imagination, isn't it interesting that you still remember this simple kindness after all these years—that you remember the person and the act so clearly? This is because the smallest kindness can be life-changing when received at the right moment.

Once, when I was only eighteen years old, I was hitchhiking through the Pacific Northwest with my backpack and a sense of adventure. After a few months I was missing my family and friends and wanted to head home. Being eighteen and not particularly good at handling money, I had barely enough cash left to feed myself on the journey home from northern Washington, all the way to Santa Cruz, California, nearly a thousand miles away. If I was lucky catching rides, I estimated I could get home with two days of constant traveling, but at the end of the second day, I was stuck by the highway for over six hours. No one would stop.

Getting stuck somewhere was not uncommon. It was still winter, and I was very cold. My face was burning from the sun and wind. My choices were to camp under an overpass or walk two miles to a tiny town and see if I could catch a Greyhound bus. If I used all of my money, meaning I wouldn't eat for twenty-four hours, I might have just enough. At the Greyhound bus station I was sad to learn I was $18 short of a ticket home. I stood speechless for a moment, then asked how far I could get with all the money I had, thinking I could hitchhike the rest of the way. As the station clerk reluctantly did the math, a middle-aged woman who had been eavesdropping stepped up and asked the clerk how much money I needed to get home. The grouchy clerk told her. As I objected, the woman ignored me and set the money down on the counter, turned, and walked out. I followed her, trying to give her back her money. She just turned back with the smile of a mother and said, "Just remember to help someone in trouble someday." I sincerely thanked her as she walked away and never forgot my promise.

About twenty-four hours later I arrived home with a little less pride, but with a new vision of kindness. I had never experienced kindness from a stranger before, and I was quite moved by it. I decided that I would look for opportunities to help others as they revealed themselves to me. Mother Teresa once said, "We can do no great things; we can do small things with great love." This woman's simple act of kindness to a stranger—who perhaps reminded her of her son or brother—took only a moment of her time and $18 (the equivalent of about $50 in today's economy). She probably doesn't even remember this event from over three decades ago, but I still remember. And I am still grateful.

Do not underestimate the power of kindness. It is a symptom of love and compassion. I believe kindness is a preeminent virtue that is born of a love for humanity. One who seeks the spiritual path but has not kindness will not walk far. Even if you have memorized the

Bible, or the Koran, the Torah, or all of the Vedas, without kindness you have achieved nothing. You have achieved only that which your laptop computer has achieved—memorization without understanding. The illiterate person who offers kindness to their fellow beings has attained more and truly embodies one of the most essential teachings of all time.

> And if I have prophetic powers, and understand all
> mysteries and all knowledge, and if I have all faith, so as to
> remove mountains, but do not have love, I am nothing.
> **—Corinthians 13:2**

Rediscovering Self-Love

In yoga, the "self" is usually defined as one of two different entities. The first is the small self, what we call the ego-mind, and the only love it really knows is narcissism, or self-admiration, and fear. But the large Self with a capital "S" is our personal soul, sometimes defined as love itself. In other words, love is our true nature. Our true essence is love itself. When we don't feel this way it is because our mind is obscured by the clouds of illusion, as storm clouds can block the light of the sun. The sun is still there, but we cannot see or feel it through the dark clouds.

So, how do we get through these dark clouds?

It is my experience from my own practice and observation as a teacher that hatha yoga clears the mind/heart of our suffering long enough for the healing emotion of gratitude to take hold again. We lose our gratitude so easily in this commerce-driven world, and take for granted our health, friendships, food, warm shelter, running water, etc. We can become so spoiled that we actually feel the universe is conspiring against us if we aren't being handed an Academy Award, or if we aren't as famous as U2.

Is it possible that we are able to love ourselves only to the degree that we have forgiven ourselves? I think if we take a look deep within ourselves with piercing honesty, we could agree that we carry around a file of our inadequacies with us—a file that contains many reasons to loathe ourselves. The result of holding anger or resentment toward ourselves is the covering of the heart center, similar to the clouds of illusion that cover the mind. Until we forgive ourselves, our hearts will remain covered—virtually imprisoned. Forgiving oneself removes these prison walls and liberates the heart. If we do not deal with the removal of this covering, we will not see joy anytime soon.

When we regain our sanity—our gratitude—the grace of life pours over us and we can find our way to self-forgiveness. This energy can be intentionally directed outward to the forgiveness of others, even eventually to our antagonists. From gratitude we can move into moments of total unconditional love and experience a blossoming beyond all radiance.

EXERCISE --
Four Steps to Rediscovering Self-Love

1) Practice your postures (asanas) with ardent focus on your breath. Breathe into your heart center; breathe in light, filling yourself; breathe out the past, that which you no longer need. If you have a spiritual practice, use your own visual image of God or name for God as you breathe in.

2) Practice gratitude. After practicing the postures with devotional breath for an hour, sit in a comfortable upright position with closed eyes. Sit quietly with a very tall spine but very relaxed shoulders. Now, bring your whole attention into your heart center and simply allow it to soften. It will soften because the heart's natural state is to be relaxed. Now, focus on someone in your personal life, someone who is indispensable to your joy, someone who instantly evokes an outpouring of gratitude. When you can feel a smile in your heart toward them, then flood them with gratitude and light.

3) Practice forgiving others. Now, focusing on this same person, flood them with forgiveness—even if you don't

think they need forgiving. Everyone needs forgiveness; pour it on them, knowing that as you let go and forgive them, as you soften your heart toward them, you will notice how the more you forgive, the more you feel forgiven. Notice that as you soften your heart toward yourself, you are softening your heart toward the entire world.

4) Practice forgiving yourself. Now ask this same being for forgiveness. Imagine them granting you sincere absolution. Now, forgive yourself. Pour this light of forgiveness onto yourself. Simply release the vise clamp on the heart. Release the past. Sit in self-forgiveness. Begin again, breathing in the energy of God as you see her/him/it—inhaling the beloved—exhaling light.

This kind of practice can lead to profound release and the rediscovering of joy. We no longer have to try and substitute fun for joy because of our lack. Joy is rightfully ours as one of the manifestations of love. Let's quit thinking about abundance. Stop asking for abundance. Instead, focus on healing, focus on gratitude, focus on forgiving; these things lead us into the state of pure love. Practice and live this way and true abundance will come, and we will love ourselves and others more deeply and joyfully.

--- •

Armor and Presence

A clenched fist cannot receive a gift, and a constrained
spirit cannot easily receive love, or even forgiveness.

Armor

Human beings tend to wear a kind of energetic, protective armor born of a fear of intimacy and designed to guard the heart from emotional pain. Our emotional armor is created mostly unconsciously for the purpose of protection, but in the end functions more like a prison cell, encaging the heart center in an attempt to protect it. This manifests as extreme feelings of isolation and loneliness. Usually, armor begins forming like scar tissue over the traumas we experienced in childhood or adolescence, but can form at any age. It manifests in our posture, body language, and facial expressions. We may have difficulty saying "I love you" to those we truly love, or hugging people meaningfully. The cumulative effect is our body telling people to keep away from us, rather than showing love and emotional accessibility. But any armor or wall designed to protect, by its very nature, also divides. And so one may go to social gatherings and wonder why no one approaches us to talk, when everything about us says "Stay away."

We might even intentionally enhance our armor by excessively lifting weights, as bodybuilders do with their massive amounts of muscle. Their armor is visible to the eye; it's a way of saying, "I'm strong and protected. Stay away from me. I'm dangerous."

Taking off our armor means to expose and reveal our spiritual heart. When we first do this we feel extremely vulnerable—and for a human being to choose to become vulnerable is a big step in our growth. We need to take off our armor long enough to see our own wounds, so then, once recognized, we can begin to heal them. If we push our wounds down, that can only last so long, just as when you have a car with a mechanical problem. When your car is making a new noise, you can pretend the problem is not there, but eventually that car will break down.

Many diseases are caused by pushing our problems down into our body, so we die early of a heart attack or get cancer. When we acknowledge our wounds, we can begin to heal ourselves; when we heal ourselves, we begin to heal everyone around us. Vulnerability does not mean passivity; it means looking at ourselves truthfully, acknowledging where we are weak and where we are strong. Just as we strengthen our outer body in our yoga practice, we also want to strengthen our internal body where it is weak, and open up where we are tight or constrained. If we do not, we will always be out of balance, and will only become more imbalanced as we get older. Taking off our armor is the beginning of transforming ourselves from silos of suffering into silos of joy.

Although yoga builds muscle, it also helps you to take the energetic armor off. For some of us, the scary part of this is that we have never had our armor off and we think, "If I take my armor off, I might get hurt. I might become too vulnerable." In actuality, what happens is that when you take your armor off, you become more approachable, more attractive and magnetic to others; you become someone people want to spend time with, as opposed to run away from. The more you choose to be authentic and allow your inner light to shine, the more you will transform from a masked stranger into a beacon of light.

It could be argued that armor has its place in life, but it's not made to sleep in, and it's not made to wear while with our loved ones. We need to learn how to consciously take it off and put it aside, perhaps eventually leaving it off forever. But many of us have worn our armor all our lives and have forgotten that we even have it on. So, perhaps we need to learn to be vulnerable and feel safe—to be emotionally exposed without feeling the threat of being ridiculed or shamed, without our status as being "strong" at stake.

Sometimes humor is also used as a kind of armor. Although we use humor ostensibly to amuse ourselves and others, when we look more closely, we can see that we often use it to simultaneously get people to like us while keeping a safe distance. Humor is often a tactic used to fill a suddenly silent dinner party, or a vulnerable moment in a conversation. Sometimes it brings us closer together, but many times it merely helps us maintain a safe distance. It's as if we want others to be charmed by us even as we want to avoid the intimacy which silence evokes. Sometimes people try so hard to be amusing, to entertain, that they make everyone around them feel unseen and unheard; nothing can be said without it being ridiculed or diminished through teasing. The joker takes center stage, and, therefore, by definition, everyone else becomes the silent, passive audience. This can end up alienating others rather than creating stronger bonds.

There is a time and a place for humor, but it is critical for the health of our relationships that we curb our every desire to be funny, or to make a pun, or to be ironic. A great deal of humor is not kind. Often our laughter is at someone else's expense. Study others as they tease and joke and you will see that this is so. Then study your own humor with an honest ear. Next time you find yourself wanting to make a joke, ask yourself, "Am I uncomfortable? Do I feel vulnerable? Is that why I want to crack a joke?" If so, then you should refrain. But if your joke comes from a place of joy and good-heartedness, then go ahead.

Humor is only one of many techniques we use to attract others. We all have little things we do to attract love. These characteristics begin when we are young. We learn to be charming, or exaggeratedly masculine or feminine, or tough, or clever, or perhaps mysterious. But I believe we are usually loved *in spite of* these things we do for love, not because of them. Usually people are not really attracted by our dance for love, but merely tolerate that part of us as a weakness. Our most beautiful and graceful power lies hidden behind these dances.

EXERCISE --
Here is a prayer you might wish to use when you want to open your heart center:

Sacred body, temple of the Divine, impermanent home
of my soul, which is who I am: I invite you to unfold, to
open, to release the armor and protection I have been
holding for so long. I now realize this armor is no longer
necessary, and it is time to flourish and blossom, to fulfill
my destiny in this lifetime—in this world. It is time to
allow all of my light, power, and mercy to shine forth,
for the benefit of my own evolution and all other sentient
beings as we move together toward the Light.

-- •

Removing the Armor

Removing our armor is done partly through breath and postures and intention, but it also takes conscious attention on our part as we move through our day. Practice being open to everyone as if they were part of your extended family. Move through your day as if it were your charge to encourage joyfulness and calm. Pay special attention to those in lower social positions and in the service industry. Address people in service positions, such as busboys, as "sir," or "miss," since they are often ignored altogether and regularly treated as slave labor. It is important for them—and for us—to treat them with extra respect. Stop and talk to the parking lot attendant; look him in the eye and thank him instead of just giving him the money and leaving, or, even worse, talking on a cell phone while in the midst of your transaction. Talking on a cell phone as you interact with others is demeaning and makes them feel like a nonentity. If your true wish is unity and transformation, this kind of behavior must cease forever. As seekers of truth, it is incumbent upon us to treat everyone with respect and care. This exercise will bring an unexpected vitality to your life, relationships, and reputation.

> *Shine brightly in your life so others of your kind may recognize you. Shine brightly in your life so others of your kind can find you from afar—through the swarm of guarded faces and flickering lives.*

Presence

The more we protect ourselves, the less we are seen; the more we reveal ourselves, the more we touch others. Saint Francis of Assisi told his followers that their task was to preach, "using words if necessary"—meaning they were to share their message with their actions and very presence.

One of the characteristics most people share is the way we underestimate our impact on the world. If you were to ask people, "Do you think that you make a difference in this world?", many would answer, "Yes, my work makes a difference." But if you then said, "No, not your work—*you*," I believe that most people would say no, believing that their presence alone has little or no impact. Most of us feel unnoticed and unseen. But each one of us, whether materially wealthy or poor, famous or obscure, has a vital and lasting impact simply through our very presence. When a person comes into contact with us, for whatever reason, we have an opportunity to better their life by simply being kind, caring, and authentic.

You are extraordinarily radiant inside; the problem is that you don't believe it. Your soul is a bright and clear light and is untarnished by your mistakes, weaknesses, and tragedies. Your soul is strong and courageous. It is wise and profoundly kind. But the insecurities of your ego-mind—or false personality—cause you to cover this radiance, and then outwardly do things and acquire things that you believe will enhance your radiance, when in fact they actually cover it up. Presence is something that is a wonderful result of your willingness to reveal your inner light, free of armor. When inward radiance is allowed to shine, people are drawn to you, no matter what your place in society, whether you live by grand or humble means.

Presence is something that is a result of a willingness to reveal your inner self, your very soul. Recall someone you know; let's say it is a young woman who works in a café. Perhaps you go to this café specifically to see her, not because of a romantic attraction, but because she is someone who brightens your day with her genuine smile each time you see her. Just to be in her presence lifts your spirit a little bit. She has no money, no economic power, no prestige—the things we are all sure we want—yet you may seek out her café even if you don't particularly like the coffee there. Why? Because she reveals her inner radiance. Then there are those you know who have the money, the power, and the connections, and yet they don't have one-tenth of the happiness of this woman at the café. When you are unafraid to share your love with others, you ennoble the world. Your open heart encourages others to open their own hearts, and what greater contribution to humanity is there?

One might argue that the young woman in the café is joyful because her life is simple, because she is young and naive, has no responsibilities, and doesn't yet know the meaning (and hardships) of "real life." This argument reinforces one of the teachings found in religions throughout the world: "Keep your life simple." Be careful that you do not bury yourself in responsibilities that are not necessary for a happy life.

It is time to stop asking for certain things or circumstances to make you happy. Why not just choose happiness, like the young woman at the little café? You might be tempted to argue that she had nothing to be happy about with no money, power, or prestige, but she chose joy nonetheless, and you find yourself drawn to her presence like a cold pilgrim to a warm fire.

Our inner stillness and joy cause people to listen, and then every time we speak we can change the world. Everyone is a child of God; everyone is born equal and has the potential of a spiritual master. Why are you always looking for someone else to save the world? Did you ever consider that it might be you? Realize that the power you seek is the power of your own soul. The peace you seek is there; the Beloved you are seeking is there. Realize this and you can exalt the world with your actions and your very presence.

EXERCISE --

Ask Yourself These Questions

1) Would you rather talk to someone who's emotionally open, or shut down?

2) Would you rather have a relationship with someone who panics and gets reactionary when things go wrong, or with someone who knows how to stay calm and positive, even amid difficulty?

3) Who would you rather live with: someone who reacts and gets stressed out at the drop of a hat, or someone who can

say, "This is tough, but it's going to be all right; we've been through things like this before," and remains positive? If this latter person is the kind you'd rather be with, chances are your partner and friends feel the same way.

--- •

Over the years I have met many people who are considered to be spiritual masters, saints, gurus, Christian leaders, and Taoist mystics. But I've only met one person whom I believe to be an enlightened being, and that was a homeless person on a dirt road in India. She was a woman in her late twenties, I do not know her name. Her health seemed remarkably vital with the exception of her stick-like legs, which were clearly withered from polio. She sat on the ground in her skirt and sweater, smiling to all, but she never asked for money. While all of the beggars I had seen up to this point reached out their hand for a contribution, she did not. Yet passersby sometimes gave her money, treating her with deference. I met her eyes and smiled, and she smiled back and said hello, apparently the only English word she knew. Then I noticed something extraordinary about this woman: She had the most joyful heart I had ever seen. Anywhere. When I met her gaze, I felt a strong and knowing feeling in my heart. She appeared to have no armor, no pride, no apparent grief or malice, but a spirit like a warm sun.

The second time I saw her I watched her from a distance for a while as I realized I had discovered an extraordinary person. I noted that most people passed her by, not noticing her, but some seemed to treat her with great respect, as if they too could see that she was very special. There she was: no social standing, withered useless legs, no money, and no hope for a husband or children. It made no logical sense to me that she was happy, no sense at all. But she was not only happy—she was also deeply joyful.

I finally walked up to her. She beamed a smile and reached her hand out to me. At first, I thought she was asking for money, but then I realized it was my hand she wanted. She sat me down next to her in the dirt and we sat together in silence. There I was, sitting in the dirt with her, holding hands. In those first moments I felt both awkward and embarrassed, and yet there I stayed. Although she was younger than I, her energy felt more like that of a wise grandmother than a young woman. Suddenly the true situation dawned on me: I felt like *I* was the unfortunate one—that I was the one being taken care of. She was the teacher and I was a new student, learning about joy and an open heart as her presence touched my soul. Tears trickled down my face as my heart cracked open. We couldn't speak the same language beyond "hello," and that was just fine.

I don't know who took care of her, but someone did, for her clothes were not tattered and her hair was clean and combed. None of it made any sense to me, but she was the happiest person I had ever met. In my observation, she seemed to have accomplished the task of removing the armor from her heart and letting her God-given essence shine forth. We have all heard axioms about money not buying happiness, but this was the most extreme example I had ever seen. She was the essence of happiness itself, and she owned nothing. None of that mattered to her. She refused to be unhappy.

And what about her effect on others? I think some viewed her as a young saint. Her heart energy, unencumbered with armor, touched strangers as they walked by—at least, those with eyes to see, as Jesus often said in the New Testament. I suspect that many people, shielded by their own armor, felt nothing; they just saw a homeless person, if they saw her at all. But those souls who were less armored were touched by her presence, and perhaps healed by it to an extent. Her open heart encouraged us to open our own hearts, and what greater contribution to humanity is there? Perhaps that is her ministry, her work in this world. Opening hearts.

After an unknown period of time, I rose and respectfully put some money in her hand, enough to take care of her for perhaps two months. The next day as I left the city to continue my journey, I looked for her to say good-bye, and to see if there was anything more I could do for her, but she was not there. I never saw her again, but her joyful presence is still with me, and I began to redefine who in life is a beggar and who is wealthy, and who deserves pity and who is a teacher.

> *We all claim to want peace, but peace is not a noun—it*
> *is a verb, which is why we cannot get it. One must live it.*
> *Peace cannot be imposed, only embodied. One cannot sell*
> *it, but one can teach it—but only by example.*

Breathing as a Spiritual Practice

> Are you looking for me? I am in the next seat. My shoulder
> is against yours. You will not find me in the stupas, not in
> Indian shrine rooms, nor in synagogues, nor in cathedrals:
> not in masses, nor kirtans, not in legs winding around
> your own neck, nor in eating nothing but vegetables. When
> you really look for me, you will see me instantly—you will
> find me in the tiniest house of time. Kabir says: Student,
> tell me, what is God? He is the breath inside the breath.
> **—Kabir, mystic poet (1398–1448)**

In our breath there is so much power to be harnessed, so much grace to be found. Many ancient languages associate breath and spirit, or breath and soul, as the same word. *Spiritus* comes from an old Latin word, meaning "to breathe," but also "soul," or "spirit." Another example is *aloha*, which originally meant "breath of God" in ancient Hawaiian. So, when we say *aloha* to each other, it essentially means "I breathe God with you." One of the translations of *Allah* means "the great breath." It seems that in many parts of the world, human beings understand the act of breathing to be much more than mere physical survival, but as an intimate connection with the divine source, and that breath is actually associated with spiritual life. In the New Testament, the word used for breath, *pneuma*, was also used for "spirit," as in "Holy Spirit."

Let's take a look at the various concepts of breath throughout the world.

Ancient Latin: *Spiritus* means "spirit" or "breath."

Ancient Greek: *Aura* literally means a "breeze" or "breath." *Pneuma* is "air," "wind," "spirit," and "breath." *Pnein* is "breathe."

Arabic: One of the translations for the name *Allah* is "The Great Breath."

Hebrew: "Breath" (*neshima*) and "soul" (*neshama*) have the same root.

German: *Atmen* in modern German means "breath." *Atman* in Sanskrit is the individual human soul, which is connected to the One Soul, or Godhead, like a bubble on the ocean.

Hawaiian: *Aloha* originally comes from two Hawaiian words— *elo*, which means the bosom, the center of the universe, and *ha*, the breath. It was originally pronounced "elo-*ha*," with the accent on the "ha." The meaning of the word is "breath of God," and the greeting is a reminder that when we breathe, we are sharing the breath of God and thus are intimately connected. (Notice the similarity of elo-ha with Elo-him, one of the Hebrew names for God.)

Chinese: *Qi* (sometimes spelled *Chi*) is translated as "life-force energy," or "breath of heaven." Breathing practice is called *Qi Gong*, "regulation of life- force energy with movement and breath."

Sanskrit: In Vedanta and hatha yoga philosophy, *prana* is life-force energy, like *Qi*. One of the main ways humans access and control this life-force energy is through the breath. In Sanskrit, *prana* is literally translated as "breath." (More specifically, to inhale is *prana*, and to exhale is *apana;* but the larger definition of *prana* is "life-force energy.")

VEDANTA: "The end of Veda," i.e., the teaching of the Upanishads, focusing on the final emancipation of the human

being from the cycle of birth, death, and rebirth. This system
of philosophy teaches that all reality is a single principle,
Brahman, and that one's goal is to transcend the limitations of
self-identity and realize one's unity with Brahman. Consistent
throughout is the exhortation that ritual be abandoned in
favor of the individual's quest for truth through meditation
governed by a loving morality, secure in the knowledge that
infinite bliss awaits the seeker. Renowned modern Vedantists
include Swami Vivekananda and Sri Aurobindo.

BRAHMAN: In the Upanishads, Brahman is the name for
the ultimate, unchanging reality, composed of pure being
and consciousness. Brahman lies behind the apparent
multiformity of the phenomenal world, and is ultimately
identical to the spiritual essence of the human being. This is a
similar ideology to the common Christian description of God
as omniscient, omnipotent, and omnipresent.

SANSKRIT: This was the classical standard language of ancient
India, and the language of the Veda, the oldest surviving
scriptures of Hinduism, dating back to around 1500 BC. Like
Latin in Europe, Sanskrit has been used by the educated
classes in India for literary and religious purposes for over two
thousand years. Although Sanskrit is now considered a dead
language, it survives even today in liturgical usage. In hatha
yoga, postures are often referred to by their Sanskrit names.

Prana and Qi; Life Force

In hatha yoga, breathing practices are called *pranayama,* or
"regulation of breath," and are born of the belief in a life-vitalizing and
life-sustaining force. This force is called *prana* and is believed to flow
through a network of fine, subtle channels called *nadis*. This is closely

related to the Chinese concept of *Qi* (or *Chi*), which flows through invisible energy channels called meridians. There is also a belief that through *pranayama* practice, one can merge with the infinite source or Godhead. Many *pranayama* practices are done while the body is sitting still, but there is also *pranayama* accompanied by movement. For example, in a vinyasa yoga class, a sequence of yoga postures led by Ujjayi breathing could be called *breath-synchronized* or *breath-initiated movement*, and is therefore one method of *pranayama*.

Qi (or *Chi*) is the Chinese word for breath. Qi Gong is an internal Chinese practice which commonly uses slow, graceful, breath-synchronized movements to promote the harmonious circulation of Qi within the human body. This is done most commonly to improve health or to heal disease, but some also practice Qi Gong more significantly to become more connected with the Tao, or God. There are Qi Gong techniques that utilize no movement, similar to *pranayama*.

> **The Tao is the breath that never dies.**
> **—Lao Tzu**

> **And Jehovah God formed man of the dust of the ground,**
> **and breathed into his nostrils the breath of life; and man**
> **became a living soul.**
> **—Genesis 2:7**

> **What is God? God is the Breath inside the breath.**
> **—Kabir**

> **All the principles of heaven and earth are living inside you.**
> **Life itself is truth, and this will never change.**
> **Everything in heaven and earth breathes.**
> **Breath is the thread that ties creation together.**
> **—Morihei Ueshiba**

Conscious Breathing

How does the way we breathe affect our stress level, health, emotions, and even our relationships? To develop the breath is to open the door to transformation. If every person in this world took ten minutes a day to practice conscious breathing, this would be a different world.

Benefits

Conscious breathing is one of the most powerful transformative tools available to us, yet even with the tremendous popularity of yoga today, it is largely untapped. People are astonished to realize they don't really know how to breathe. Of course everyone reading this right now is inhaling and exhaling, but it doesn't mean that they're breathing in a way that's going to significantly impact them.

Here are some of the health benefits of conscious breathing:

- Stronger lungs with vastly increased capacity
- A healthier heart and stronger diaphragm
- In many cases, the ability to heal asthma and also release the habit of smoking
- The nervous system is calmed, diminishing stress, lowering one's blood pressure and heart rate, and thereby improving sleep and maintaining a more-enhanced mental state while awake
- Enables us to identify and heal emotional wounds from our past

Making breathing practices a part of your daily life will initiate meaningful transformation much more deeply and profoundly than yoga postures alone. Not that the practice of postures isn't extremely significant, but if you have a posture practice and still breathe unconsciously, your mind/nervous system is probably still restless. What are the signs of a restless mind? Trouble sleeping or grinding your jaw at night, addictions, anger issues, anxiety, acting out, and what is commonly (but, I believe, mistakenly) called ADD (attention deficit disorder).

People who have a dedicated breathing practice generally experience far fewer of these symptoms. Symptoms? Yes; what you may think of as personality traits may be more accurately called symptoms. Most people know that our inner state is determined by heredity, upbringing, diet, environment, and stress; but our inner state can also be affected or even controlled by our intentions, will, and conscious practices. For example, we know that alcohol and other legal and illegal drugs can calm us down, but what most people don't realize is that the nervous system can be brought into harmony through breathing techniques, and with zero side effects.

Our emotions are so powerful that until they are healed and brought back into balance, we cannot go far on our transformational journey. Think of the horses pulling the carriage in that ancient analogy: If the horses are reactionary and highly skittish or aggressive, they cannot be tamed and trained to pull the carriage forth on the soul's journey. So, through the techniques put forth in this system—the practice of gratitude, forgiveness, breathing techniques, etc.—we can heal ourselves on the emotional level.

Many people believe they are not in need of emotional healing, mistakenly believing that their health symptoms, such as chronic sleep disorders, depression, anxiety, overeating, and smoking tobacco, are issues of the mind or body, but not emotionally rooted. Therefore, many become inexplicably stuck on their path, not from lack of effort, but because of the chains of the past known as anger, grief, and fear. These buried emotions, like thorns in the heart, can be crippling to our spiritual practice. It is as simple as this: When we are in pain, we become self-centered and myopic. When we heal, we become more empathetic, selfless, and sympathetic to the pain and welfare of others. We also become more sensitive to subtle energies and are able to hear the inner voice of our intuition, previously drowned out by the noise within.

The Impact of Breathing on Our Relationships

Emotional healing with breath has a powerful impact on our relationships because when we are carrying emotional wounds inside of us, we tend to hurt the people we love the most. These wounds are invisible to the untrained eye. The ego, our false personality, covers our heart like a dark blanket covering a lamp. When we breathe deeply and consciously, the ego dissipates, uncovering the heart center. Then, like the sunrise, what was dark becomes illuminated with the light from our own heart, and this light shines brightly in all areas of our life.

The ramifications of this are profound. Show me a student with a powerful and refined breathing practice, and I'll show you a person undergoing rapid transformation. Your very life changes quickly as your breath melts the ego, almost as fire melts ice. Your heart center opens wider, and so do your eyes, and then you then see differently and make new choices based on this new vision. When this happens you will begin to sense your purpose and veer toward your true path. Others will also begin to sense your purpose as well, so you will have guides to point the way toward your destiny. These guides may be friends or strangers, and by grace you will find them as your living signposts.

How It Works

The first concept we need to understand is that our breath and our emotions are interrelated. We speak of them as two things, but they are really not. We all know this instinctively. We know that when we have extreme physical pain, we unconsciously, without any training, start trying to regulate deep breathing because we know subconsciously that it helps to decrease pain. Somehow we also seem to know innately that it can help us to deal with strong emotions such as fear and rage. For childbirth, an event often accompanied by intense bodily pain, women are offered breathing classes to help them learn to relax through the pain and to diminish the level of fear. So, physical and emotional pain are both affected by the breath, and can be managed or regulated with breathing techniques.

But how could it possibly be that simply breathing in and out in a particular way can change the way we feel or think? What does manipulating the body have to do with how we feel?

Here is an example: Let's say you've received very upsetting news, and consequently, your neck and shoulders begin to stiffen and become very uncomfortable. Sound familiar? When you get emotionally upset, your body gets upset too, and it tenses and contracts; your breath becomes shallow and erratic as the body starts to respond to your emotional state, because, again, your body and emotions are not separate. Now, let's say a body worker massages your tight muscles. Then what happens? You feel better—not just your shoulders, but inwardly, emotionally, as well. It's the tail wagging the dog. By soothing the body, the emotions and the mind are also soothed. I think massage is one of the most interesting and overlooked miracles in life. We live in our bodies and we store our emotions in them. We call it stress, but that's inaccurate; , it's not just stress, we actually store our emotions in different parts of our body. The fact that another human being can put their hands on us and take the pain away is truly a miracle.

Now, conversely, when you feel happy and inspired, your body also feels happy and inspired. You get a spring in your step. Somebody who's really joyful stands and walks completely differently than does someone who is depressed because the body and the emotions are interconnected. As above—so below.

According to traditional Chinese medicine (acupuncture), different internal organs of the body actually are in relation with different specific emotions. Which emotions would you say are contained in the lungs? What happens to the lungs when you become very sad? What do they do? They spasm. You start to cry and the lungs convulse. Most of us never really stop to think about it, but the idea of sobbing is quite amazing. You can be sitting in a normal state, and then you get some sad news and your lungs go into spasm, water comes out of your eyes, and the body goes into a completely new state. Your stomach and liver do not go into spasm, but when you start to cry, your lungs do. We have named this "sobbing." So it is obvious that the lungs express our grief, but they also express our inspiration. The two emotions that the lungs contain, store, and express, according to Chinese medicine, are grief and inspiration. Inspiration is when we suddenly take a fast, deep inhale and say, "Look who's here!" The word *inspire* is Latin, meaning "to breathe in."

"Aahh! I've got an idea! I'm so excited!" This comes with an inhale. We respond to sadness, despair, and loss with an exhale. The Latin word *expiration* means "to breathe out." It also means to pass away in the medical world.

Why are some of us afraid to breathe deeply?

Many of us have fear about breathing deeply because we know deep down that our breath is somehow connected to our emotions. If we are stressed out and besieged with unexpressed grief, rage, or fear, then deep breathing terrifies us. So, we keep our breaths small and shallow and erratic, no matter how many times our yoga teacher tells us to breathe deeply. Like opening Pandora's Box, we feel that if we took a deep breath, our life might fall apart. But the inverse is true. When we take a deep breath, we fall deeper into life.

I have taught workshops in smaller, rural towns, and, generally speaking, getting a class to breathe deeply takes very little effort on my part. Whereas in major cities where stress is prevalent, and especially in New York City, getting a class to commit to deep breathing is like pulling teeth. This is because in contemporary urban life, there is so much stress, so much competitiveness, and so much frozen energy around people's hearts; transforming this to a new healthy state is a huge leap. For some, opening the chest is the hardest part of one's yoga practice because it is in the chest that we keep our grief and our old memories, and to open the chest would mean dealing with a new personality and a new life—a massive transformation. This is what we simultaneously strive for and fear. It is like we are stepping on the accelerator and the brake pedal at the same time.

So when we do deep-breathing exercises, we access our buried emotions and they rise to the surface. Our first reaction, again, may be fear of losing control and releasing a never-ending river of tears. But if we persevere, we may discover that the experience not only doesn't destroy us, but that it will actually liberate us from the prison of our past. We begin to feel like we are releasing a great weight off of our chest. You've heard the old saying, "Get it off your chest"?

Sometimes our repressed emotions involve pain or trauma from our childhood. The trauma may have been so profound that it will take a very long time to heal, even with therapy, particularly for those who have been sexually or physically abused as children. But for most of us, our early experiences of pain—such as being neglected, bullied, or shamed—although very real, are not as extreme. As children we often had no way of processing our emotions, so, not knowing what else to do, we repressed them. Then, as adults, we habituated pushing down our emotions, eventually forgetting they were even there.

Perspective

Something that was monstrously huge at five years old is not so huge when you're an adult. (I am not referring to physical or sexual abuse.) For example, as an adult, everything seems so small when you go back and visit your childhood home. The vast open field behind your house is really just a city lot. You see the tree that you fell from long ago, and the branch that seemed like it was fifty feet from the ground was really only five feet high. Similarly, with some past emotional events we still feel like we're children because we haven't dealt with these issues since we were small, so, we have considerable fear of going back into these unresolved ordeals. The grief linked to these issues—which we repress in the chest region, to a certain extent—can separate us from the very ones we love, because it's hard to embrace someone who's living behind a wall, or armor. We must always remember that any wall erected to protect also divides.

As previously mentioned, I experienced a great deal of physical pain when I was a young child from five orthopedic surgeries, several broken bones, and months spent in plaster casts. I learned to accept this pain, cope with it, and tolerate it. The negative side of this is I also unknowingly trained myself to ignore it. Ignoring pain in a crisis can be useful, but as a habit, it is not. It caused me to disassociate not only from feelings of physical pain but also emotional pain as well. Later, as a young adult, I came to regard my feet as mostly a "problem area," and virtually ignored them as opposed to trying to nurture and heal them.

At age twenty-one, I had my first session with a professional body worker. When she had finished working on my back and moved to my feet, it was a memorable moment for me. Up until that time, no one had ever touched my feet in a caring or loving manner, including myself. My mother had dutifully and with great care looked after me during my surgeries and so on, in ways I am deeply grateful for, but she did not or would not hold or massage my feet, even when I was an infant. When the body worker massaged my feet, I felt tremendous emotions swelling up in me from this closed-off area of my body, and I think that it was the beginning of a long healing for me.

After the bodywork session, I felt quite liberated and raw, simply from someone touching my feet with kindness. I believe that subconsciously I had always feared thinking about (and, especially, feeling) my feet because they had been a source of pain for so long. So, I had disassociated myself from them for fear of more pain, and also, because of shame. I was ashamed of my strange-looking feet that had caused my parents so much trouble and money. But, like the boy who went back home and saw that the tree branch was only five feet from the ground (rather than fifty), I discovered that by exploring the feelings in my feet, instead of perpetuating trauma, I experienced healing. I was an adult and could now process emotions in a way that I could not as a little boy. Once realizing this, I was able to choose to continue healing my feet and the emotional wounds they held, and this, of course, healed more than my feet; it also helped to heal my relationships with myself and others.

When we repress emotional pain, where does the pain go? To a large extent it stays in our bodies. It is like we use our body as a cork in a bottle. This can create two kinds of very serious consequences: First, disease. Many people, chiefly in alternative medicine, believe that unexpressed or unresolved grief can create ailments over time, and even deadly diseases such as cancer. Cancer and heart disease do not just have to do with heredity and cholesterol levels. For instance, with heart disease, research has indicated that a man who has a wife who loves him is less likely to die of heart disease than one who doesn't.

Some studies reveal that trapped or repressed negative feelings increase a person's level of cortisol, often referred to as the "stress hormone," which has been found to directly suppress immune system functioning. When the immune system is not functioning properly, cancer cells that exist in every human being can multiply and form tumor sites. Remember: The body, emotions, and mind are not separate. If we stuff our emotions down into our body, the emotions can, in their way, fester, and then can literally become illness, then disease, and then finally a cause of premature death.

Second, unexpressed emotional pain can destroy our relationships. We tend to hurt the people we love the most when we are carrying emotional wounds. Unresolved resentments lodge deep in our heart like thorns.

Imagine someone with open wounds under their clothes. You can't see these wounds because they are covered, but sometimes when you hold them, their reaction is like a wounded animal. They lash out because you have unknowingly touched their wounds beneath their clothing. Even if we cover up our wounds, they're still there. As the people we love get close enough to us, they will unintentionally but inevitably touch our wounds, and we will unintentionally but inevitably lash out, possibly doing great harm to the relationship.

The Impact of Parents

If you were raised in a house where one of your parents often dwelled in a negative state of mind, the whole house felt it. Dad or Mom came home in a terrible mood, and the kids would start walking on eggshells. It infected the whole house like poison. Conversely, when that parent came home in a great mood, calm and cheerful, this also affected the whole household. You went up to your dad or your mom and they smiled and hugged you, and you would feel loved and safe. People go to therapy every day, voicing how they wish their parents were like that. Imagine if your parents had taken ten minutes each day outside in the hall or on the porch and did breathing exercises before coming into the house in order to bring their emotions into balance. How much would that have affected your life?

Now the shoe is on the other foot; *we* are the adults. We are the ones coming home carrying the stress in our bodies. Is there value in us being able to heal ourselves so that we are not the stressed-out parent invading the house instead of living in it? Is there value in being able to heal ourselves so that we are not the one to fly off the handle over silly things when we could just smile instead? Breathing practices can change your life because they change your behavior, and even the choices you make, and that affects all of your relationships and can alter the course of your destiny.

Grief Is Stored in the Lungs

One of the ways many people push grief down in the lungs is through smoking cigarettes, or marijuana. I have discussed the relationship between breath and cigarette smoking with several acupuncturists. They often say something to this effect: "We call cigarette smokers 'fire-breathers.' Smoking is a way of pushing the emotions down. Have you noticed that people almost always start smoking at around age twelve or thirteen, during puberty? It's a way for young people who don't know how to deal with their feelings to sublimate or repress their problems."

Most people do take up smoking as adolescents, when, not so coincidentally, there are so many new and difficult emotions and hormones to deal with. Life at home and at school can be challenging, and the young teen may discover that they can emotionally "self-medicate" to a degree with cigarettes. It's a way of pushing the emotions down and keeping them at bay. The hot smoke goes into the moist lungs and tamps the grief down, and at the same time gives them a little nicotine boost of perceived power. But of course what they do not realize is that the emotions are not gone, just stored away, and that this method of repressing them will have its consequences in the future.

The energies of the lungs are partly about survival of the physical body, according to Chinese medical theory. When the physical body is in perceived turmoil, unless the individual has a great support system to manage their painful emotions, they may fall prey to smoking to help them endure. This phenomenon is evident with soldiers in war. The percentage of soldiers in combat who smoke is extremely high, perhaps because they experience so much trauma. According to the Center for Tobacco Research and Intervention at the University of Wisconsin School of Medicine and Public Health, about 50 percent of soldiers deployed to Iraq return addicted to tobacco. Cigarettes are no longer included in soldiers' rations as they were during World War I and World War II.

If you've ever managed to stop smoking after much effort and then three or four years later you started up again, you know very well what caused it. It wasn't a billboard promoting cigarettes, or a magazine ad, and it wasn't somebody saying, "Here, have a cigarette." It was a new tragedy. It was a broken heart or a rejection, such as losing your job or having to deal with sudden loss. The emotions start coming up again and you reach for something that's tried and true—something that you feel will help you subdue the intense and newly emerging emotions. Many quit smoking only to start up again years later because of something like this.

In my yoga classes I emphasize breathing as a central feature, and I never ask people to stop smoking. They have plenty of people in their life doing that; they don't need one more. I just teach them to breathe and breathe and breathe. And then eventually most of them will come to me and say with a smile, "You know what? I stopped smoking three months ago." This is a natural result of learning to breathe well.

Ocean Breathing

Practicing ocean breathing is a fundamental tool for taking off one's armor and opening the heart center for emotional healing. To breathe here now helps us to be here now. When and how often should we practice?

To insert ocean breathing practice into your everyday life, I recommend that first, if you practice yoga in a class setting, that you make your practice *breath-centric*. Don't go anywhere without your breath. Every movement should be initiated by an inhale or exhale. Second, I recommend that you practice ocean breathing for ten minutes at least once per day. This can be done at any time of day as long as it is an hour or more after eating. If you can, practice upon rising in the morning and again in the evening, even just before going to bed. Breathing fresh air is obviously advisable if possible, so step outside or practice near an open window. If access to fresh air is not possible, do your practice anyway. I practice on international flights where the air quality is dismal at best, and feel much better for doing so. You may notice that your pets seem to enjoy your breathing practice, and your young children will too.

The ocean breathing exercise, which sounds like the ocean's waves coming to the shore and going back out again, enlivens the lungs and expands them, dynamically pulling in fresh air (*prana*) and then expelling stale air and stress (*apana*). It is known for calming the mind and can also be very effective for helping to process grief.

> In the yoga world, ocean breathing is traditionally called Ujjayi breathing (pronounced oo-JAH-yee), and is the most common breath used in hatha yoga practice. I call it ocean breathing because it sounds like the tide, and because it is more easily remembered and less likely to intimidate beginners.

Instructions for Ocean Breathing

Stand in a comfortable spot. Look down at your feet and separate them by about three feet. Make sure they are straight.

Now, as you bend your knees about six inches, lengthen your spine up toward the ceiling.

Bring your hands to the heart center; press them together gently as if in prayer.

Now, from here, inhale through your mouth as you move your arms straight out to the sides at shoulder height—arms open, elbows slightly bent. Pause, and then exhale them back to the heart.

Inhale and open the arms again. Then bring your hands back to prayer position, exhaling audibly through your mouth just as if you were fogging a mirror with your warm breath. Continue the same movements with your arms as you breathe this way, making the "fogging the mirror" sound on both the inhale and the exhale. Your mouth stays open continuously and the lips should not purse together. Remember to breathe into the sides of your ribs.

Continue for five minutes and work up to ten. (I recommend using a timer so you are not distracted by time.)

You may experience an emotional feeling or even some tears after practicing this breath. If that happens, simply receive it as a healing experience. Afterward you'll feel refreshed and peaceful.

Review:

Make the sound of fogging the mirror with your breath.

Keep a straight, enlivened spine but keep your knees slightly bent.

Relax the shoulder blades downward.

Broaden the chest and remember to breathe into the sides of your ribs.

Keep mouth open, teeth apart. Do not purse your lips or use them to breathe.

Should I do ocean breathing through my mouth or through my nose?

I teach ocean breathing with the inhale and exhale both through the open mouth, lips apart, relaxed and never pursed. It is significantly more efficient to teach it this way. People become very confused trying to understand how to make the ocean sound with the mouth closed, while everyone has already produced the sound by fogging a mirror or their sunglasses to clean them. Also, with the mouth open, the sound level is substantially louder, so the student can hear the subtleties of the breathing much better. This of course improves their technique. Then, once a student can do ocean breathing very adeptly (which usually takes doing the exercise at least ten times), then I teach them to breathe making the same sound in the same way, but doing so with the lips closed and the teeth slightly apart. The method of producing the ocean-like sound is identical; the only change is the closing of the lips. In conclusion, mouth-open variation is called level one, and mouth-closed variation, level two.

Safety Note

If you become dizzy, stop the exercise and bend over, lowering your head below your heart; the flush of blood to the head prevents fainting. Then lie down until you feel ready to stand again.

Resistance to breathing is resistance to change. Resistance to change is resistance to living. Resistance to living is a kind of walking death. Inhale deeply, friend; inhale. Your breathing practices and emotional healing will lead you to virtuous behavior and a life of non-grasping and joy. The heart, unencumbered by grief and resentment, will blossom from merely an emotional heart into a spiritual heart.

Can breathing be done while sitting in a chair?

Ocean breathing can be done while sitting in a chair or a wheelchair. It can also be utilized with your meditation by breathing a little softer and not including the arm movement.

Here are some fundamental and practical breathing techniques to help get you started.

How to Do Ocean Breathing while Sitting:

The first thing you need is to be able to sit with your spine straight. You can sit on a straight-backed chair, preferably without leaning against the backrest, or you may sit cross-legged on folded-up blankets or a firm cushion on the floor.

If while sitting cross-legged your knees look higher than your hips, place some more blankets or some kind of bolster beneath your buttocks to elevate your hips higher than the knees. This will allow you to sit more comfortably on the floor, achieving a straighter spine and making your breathing more efficient. It is important that you be able to sit on the floor without feeling like you're tipping over backwards.

Now, slump down for a moment. Collapse the upper spine and concave the chest, like when you sit in front of the computer. Now, while staying in this position, take a deep breath. See how it feels. It doesn't work so well, does it? Your lungs feel like little walnuts. Now, sit up very straight and take a deep breath. Feel the difference?

For this reason alone we need to sit up straight to breathe well, because just on a very functional, practical level, the spine needs to be straight in order for the lungs to be able to expand and contract freely.

So, again, make certain that your hips are level or higher than your knees. Lift your spine and rest your hands on your thighs or knees, palms facing up. Do not allow your chest and shoulders to collapse forward.

Review:
> Sit tall.
> Keep a straight, enlivened spine.
> Relax the shoulders downward.
> Broaden the chest.

While you breathe deeply, try expanding your chest on every inhale. The reason is that the chest is the most difficult area of the body to open. You may think, "No, my hamstrings are the tightest." But, in fact, for most people the region of the heart is energetically the tightest area. I don't necessarily mean tight muscularly, but rather, emotionally constricted. This is the area we protect. This area, the upper trunk or chest region, is called the thorax, which means "shield" in Latin. Our vernacular is filled with metaphors for feeling powerful emotions in the thorax. "She broke my heart"; "He stabbed me in the back," etc. So, this is the area where the emotional healing work needs to be done.

The Three-Minute Breath

What you'll need:

- A timer or stopwatch
- Your cell phone turned off
- Some folded-up blankets or a straight-backed chair to sit on

Benefits:

This exercise slows down time and you will begin to feel clear and calm. It also establishes the ability to stay with one-pointed focus due to the act of counting your breaths.

How to do it:

Sit as described in the previous exercise. Now, for the next three minutes, you're going to sit up tall and count your breaths and think of nothing else. Use ocean breathing for this exercise and keep track of the time with your timer or stopwatch. Do not hold your breath for more than two seconds at the top of each inhale and bottom of each exhale. The Three-Minute Breath is not a retention holding exercise; it's very slow breathing, counting your breaths—that's all.

To prepare, exhale. Now, begin breathing in, counting your breaths. I suggest you do this with your eyes closed. Count your breaths. There's no right amount. It doesn't matter what the number is. Sit upright and count your breaths. See if you can stay focused for three minutes.

Once you are finished, try to remember what the number was for next time. For most people it's somewhere between six and thirty breaths in three minutes. Eventually, you will be able to breathe one breath in three minutes: one inhale for a minute and a half, one exhale for a minute and a half. But the point is not to train yourself to breathe one breath in three minutes so you can brag to your friends; the aim of slowing the breath down to that extent is for the calming and focusing benefits to the mind and nervous system. Most important, the soul becomes aware of itself.

Tears in Resting Pose

When you learn to breathe well, at times you will inevitably experience tears. This is caused by the releasing of trapped grief that you've been holding onto for years. Personally, when I started practicing yoga and breathing deeply, each day at the end of class I'd lie down and I'd have a few tears trickling down my face. I wasn't weeping, but I'd have some tears and I'd feel that little spasm the lungs do when we are about to cry. One day I took the teacher aside; I was embarrassed, but I told him what was happening, hoping for an explanation. Unfortunately, he wasn't very knowledgeable on this subject and he said he didn't know. For nearly a year, at the end of almost every class I'd have tears trickling down my face. Then one day I noticed that there were no more tears.

Eventually I met a teacher who understood this phenomenon, and she said, "Oh yeah, of course—that's what happens. And has it stopped yet?" I said, "Yes, it hardly ever happens anymore." Then she said, "That means it took you about one year to get the old grief out of your body. It doesn't mean that you're not going to have new grief, because this is life, but you've gotten the old grief out."

It began to makes sense to me because I found my behavior was changing; I was becoming a more relaxed and happy person.

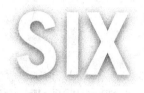

The Third Pillar—The Body

We know this body of flesh, blood, and bone is a temporary vehicle, but for the time being, this vehicle is our temple, and our ability to live a spiritually based and emotionally healthy life (not to mention a longer life) is significantly reliant on high-level health and vitality. If we want to really transform our life into what it is meant to be and realize any meaningful goals beyond the short term, we must first fulfill the most basic principle: control of the body.

Our body is commonly treated as something that carries our brain around, or something that our hands stick out of, doing things for us—basically, a brain holder and a hand station. We don't really notice the body unless it hurts, craves food, wants sex, or won't fit into its clothes anymore. There's no real sense of living in the body. Some may think, "Well, so what?" But then they wonder why their body has chronic pain, why they don't sleep well, or why they grind their teeth at night. Sometimes we just don't connect the dots.

Healing Yourself

In the Western world, most people do not see a connection between their spiritual life and their bodies. For example, a person may go to church and then play a game of tennis, treating the two activities as completely separate and unrelated events. In fact, we have two categories in our vernacular for them: one is sacred, the other athletic, or fun—as if the body is not part of our spiritual life whatsoever.

Then, as we age, most of us just let our bodies fall apart. Many watch sports avidly but don't participate in them; in fact, in America, 40 percent of us don't exercise at all. We even fuel the fire by abusing our bodies with negligent and compulsive eating habits, and then when we inevitably become ill from this neglect, we turn to God and pray desperately for a miraculous healing. What we do not realize, sadly, is that we are asking God to rescue us from afflictions we could have prevented on our own with different behavior, and could still quite possibly heal by taking action. The American Medical Association admits that over 60 percent of health problems in the United States could be prevented with simple actions and good habits. So, the disconnect is, when it comes to feeding and exercising the body, we don't think of God or our spirituality at all, but when it comes to curing our body of significant illness and disease, then we turn to God for help.

The ancient yogis said that the breath was our direct energetic connection to spirit, or God. If this is so, then if you focus on your breath with spiritual devotion, hatha yoga becomes a spiritual practice, a wordless prayer. This is because as you fill your body/mind with breath, you are also filling yourself with spirit and the breath of God. Your body then radiates who you are from your soul, and what you stand for in this world. So, if you desire it, your spiritual life and your body can be brought together as one. Instead of solely following a health regime, it also becomes a prayer regime, and, as a side effect, vibrant health is yours.

EXERCISE --

Look at and identify your biggest challenges with your own body, and how your actions, or lack of action, ultimately create not only physical challenges, but also emotional wounds as well—wounds such as shame and self-loathing. Let's say that overeating is your biggest challenge/wound.

You know that it is your own hand that feeds this wound, one spoonful at a time, creating suffering. The wonderful news is that you also have the power to heal this wound by your own hand, unlocking the prison door and releasing yourself, and that's something to rejoice in and then act on.

--- •

The Wild Horse

The body, like a wild horse, must at times be coaxed, loved, rewarded, and sometimes tricked until it trusts and obeys you, and then, like a tamed stallion, it will allow you to ride it, subjecting its own will to yours. Without accomplishing this, the body will plague you with unyielding desires and the ruinous consequences of those lusts, including eating disorders, constant cravings (for sex, alcohol, cigarettes, sugar, caffeine, fat), and then insomnia, headaches, a compromised immune system, constipation, restlessness, anxiety, and depression. And that is just the beginning; after these come the giants of illness: cancer, diabetes, heart disease, and so on—all because we cannot say no when we should, even if it kills us slowly and painfully. If one truly desires to rise to greatness, to transform, even to know God, one must first control the body. With rare exceptions, there is no escaping this fact.

Hatha Yoga—The Path of Action

As we all know, no matter how physically fit we are, no matter how rich or successful we are, no matter how smart we are, we are still subject to mental and emotional turmoil, anxiety, and depression. Even worse, when we succumb to these negative emotions, we pull our family and even our community down with us. But the good news is that the converse is also just as true.

Hatha yoga is a profound evolutionary system that will benefit everyone who has the passion to change his or her troubled existence into an extraordinary life. It has changed my life forever, and every day I see it transform more and more people into happier, healthier, and more empowered beings.

When we dedicate one hour a day to becoming better human beings while simultaneously improving our health, we elevate not only our own lives, but also the life of our entire community. Hatha yoga is a system for:

- healing, physically and emotionally;
- accelerating our personal evolution; and
- setting a direction of higher consciousness and kindness in our relationships and the world.

There are many people who just practice the postures without any of these internal aspects; while they do get stronger and more flexible, they are often still unhappy and depressed. So, they become strong, flexible, depressed people rather than stiff, weak, depressed people. You need to focus equally on your internal life, and not allow yourself to believe it will fix itself. Connect the dots.

Whatever your body/mind applies itself to and improves on in your daily yoga practice will be applicable to the outside world as well. When you improve your attention span in the yoga room, it doesn't stay in the room; it leaves with you and will be applied to anything else you do—your work, your conversations, your relationships . . . everything. When you learn to deliberately calm your nervous system in your yoga practice, you will find yourself doing the same inner practice throughout your day. The body begins to be more at ease, storing less negative anxiety and tension; this cumulatively alters your demeanor to that of a more relaxed and patient person.

Sometime I hear people say, "I can't do yoga; I'm not very good at it." This usually translates as, "I am stiff." Remember, yoga is not merely flexibility and postures.

Imagine two people practicing side by side. One is stiff and struggling in a posture, barely able to open up his hips, struggling away, but he is not letting it bother him. Instead, he feels calm in this difficult moment, centered in deep breathing.

Then there is a second person next to him, able to wrap his legs around his neck, but breathing erratically, thinking negative thoughts. Whose practice is better? Flexibility is not the aim; it is a side effect. The postures are the raft to get you to the other side of the river. This is not a competition in boating. We want to get to the other side of the river—that is the aim. If you find joy and you are living a meaningful life, then you are becoming good at yoga.

Most come to yoga to heal their body—their lower back, their knees, and so on—and it works, but that's not what keeps them returning year after year. They come back because yoga heals their *lives*. When we enthusiastically tell our friends and family how yoga has changed our lives, we may get bewildered stares or even a derisive look at the idea that what they assume is merely stretching exercises could possibly have such a grand impact. Then they are certain you have joined a cult. This is because they do not have any idea that yoga could be anything more than stretching our hamstrings.

To the novice, yoga appears to be primarily physical, and it's often misunderstood as such. From a cursory glance, it appears to be merely a practice of moving the body in and out of postures, but this is a conclusion of great error. Imagine a person who could not read, and had never even heard of a book. Now imagine this person coming upon someone on a park bench reading a life-changing novel. The illiterate person would only see a woman on a bench, staring at a box-shaped object, sitting very still and apparently doing absolutely nothing. This is because he cannot see within the reader's mind and heart and experience what the reader is experiencing. Similarly, if someone who knew nothing of yoga peeked through the window of a yoga school, they would see what might appear to be "just a stretching class." Because of the observer's background in sports or dance, this would be a reasonable assumption. But again, this assumption would be far from accurate. The ultimate power of yoga lies beyond what the eyes can see.

As previously covered, conscious breathing combined with the various yoga postures is healing and harmonizes your nervous system. It is this transformation of the nervous system that affects great change in your life, because it begins to alter your decision-making process. This is how it works: A calm and centered person makes different decisions than a stressed person does. An angry person chooses differently than a joyful one. When the nervous system is harmonized, we begin to resonate with calmer people and places. We slowly discover that we don't need such intense stimuli to feel alive, so we let go little by little, almost unconsciously, of negative habits, foods, and substances. We need fewer stimuli yet feel more alive. These apparently small changes accumulatively redirect the course of our life. We find ourselves on a new road, and are astonished at how it all happened.

> *Remember, the goal is not to tie ourselves in knots—we're already tied in knots. The aim is to untie the knots in our heart. The aim is to unite with the ultimate, loving, and peaceful power of the universe and fully awaken into the highest level of human consciousness.*

EXERCISE --
Commit to a hatha yoga practice six days a week, even if it is only for forty minutes a day. Forty minutes a day, for yourself, for your family, for the rest of your life.

-- •

SportsLogic vs. YogaLogic

John Lennon once said, "Life is what happens to you while you're making other plans." Consider that yoga is what happens to you while you think you're trying to get into shape.

The term *SportsLogic* applies especially to Type A personalities. In sports we are taught to sacrifice our body in order to win; in yoga, we are taught to sacrifice our ego in order to transform.

In the industrial world, we are told from an early age to push ourselves to the limit, to compete on every level. The jobs we try for include the maxim "must be able to work under pressure." But every day the pressure on our body, heart, and our nervous system builds and builds.

Common Tactics Taught in Business and Sports
- Endure
- Force
- Intimidate
- Dominate
- Win

Since these methods are sacraments in business and sports, it is understandable that many people try and use the same methods in their yoga practice. But hatha yoga, although it also uses the body as a tool, has a different aim, and that is to develop things that can never be taken away—even after the death of the body. The aim is to awaken from a kind of sleepwalking state that we call ordinary life and to remember who and what we truly are, cultivating and opening our heart center. Opening our heart center releases and cultivates a conscious energy that we call love. When we are in a state of love, we are happy, and those we come into contact with will feel happy as well. The ancient sages say that this is why we are here. It is by opening this center that we find joy and true empowerment.

Most actions people take each day are in pursuit of joy and empowerment. Every choice we make regarding entertainment, food, sex, media—it is all for joy and empowerment. It is as if we want to walk around the globe to get to the spot directly behind us, instead of just turning around. Opening the heart center is turning around, and it is the beginning of a meaningful life.

A few years before I began teaching, I was acquainted with a woman who had practiced hatha yoga for decades. She had naturally limber joints and was flexible and quite strong as well. Although I was impressed with her physical practice, I noticed that her disposition was a bit anxious and critical of other people, and this confused me. I didn't understand how someone with such an advanced yoga practice could carry such nervous energy, anxiousness, and negativity. As I became more aware of the significance of breath during yoga practice, I realized that during yoga, this woman's breathing was in fact inaudible. Upon closer observation, I realized her breathing was quite shallow and even tense. Her rib cage barely moved.

Then I comprehended why she never seemed to sweat even though she practiced very hard: She wasn't utilizing Ujjayi breathing, and was therefore building no internal heat. The picture became a little clearer. One day, she confided to me that she had begun wearing a retainer to pull in her front teeth. It turned out that when she practiced yoga, she would unconsciously press her tongue into her upper front teeth with such force that she had changed the angle of her bite. She now needed a retainer to realign her teeth. This explained her condition to me. In her dutiful practice of strength, flexibility, and apparent will, she had unknowingly been cultivating internal tension. Her breath was shallow, meaning that it would gather and then "freeze-dry" this tension within. This is why she could practice daily and still be "a bit high-strung," as she described herself.

The fact that none of her teachers had apparently dealt with this issue of hers years before elucidates my opinion that most yoga teachers in America do not know how to teach breathing as a priceless part of a yoga practice.

Conclusion: A good posture practice alone produces better health, strength, and flexibility, i.e., certain health and athletic benefits. But a practice of postures combined with a devoted breathing practice will open the lungs and release old grief from the chest and shoulders and hips, calming the nervous system and causing the storm within the mind to begin to recede.

Learn to abandon the competitive mind-set. Study your own tendency toward SportsLogic and notice what it brings out in you. Then, if you are convinced it isn't helping you to get where you truly want to be, examine YogaLogic as an alternative and see what happens. *Remember, it doesn't matter how deep into a posture you go—what does matter is who you are when you get there.*

-- •

Where We Hold Emotions in the Body

Nothing happens in the mind that doesn't happen in the body. They are one. Within our bodies we hold the mental, emotional, and tactile experiences of our past and present. In some teachings it is believed the body even contains the quintessence of our former lifetimes, and that we manifest these inherent tendencies (called *samskaras* in Sanskrit) through our character and ultimately our behavior. By manipulating the body with hatha yoga, we release buried negative emotions that are crippling to our spiritual progress, and we guide the crooked course of our inherent tendencies straight—like the tail wagging the dog. Our spiritual intent realigns our misaligned emotional body.

From my experience as a practitioner, and especially as a teacher, I have witnessed that certain areas of the body contain different emotions. Every week I see entire classes of students collectively responding to the same postures in very similar, even predictable ways.

The Face

The face creates a mask of a person's dominant and pervasive emotions, such as an angry face, a sad expression, or an expression of chronic disappointment. You can observe this particularly on people over forty-five years old, as lines develop that are visible to the world. Most of us think of this as a cosmetic problem, but what the lines tell us is how we have responded emotionally to our life thus far. A person's everyday mask does not reveal their pervasive emotion, but as the face hardens over decades, these emotions come to the surface and are revealed. We seldom see this mask because when we look into the mirror, we change our expression to our "mirror face." This could explain why so many of us don't like candid photos taken, because in the mirror we do not see ourselves the way we look in reality.

One simple technique to transform this negative habit into a positive one is to add the act of relaxing your face on your list that you use for postures. In other words, when you go into a posture, you have a list—things to think about and adjust, and usually in a particular order. In Downward Facing Dog, for instance, you might first think about the placement of your feet, then your hands, then the quality of your breath, then the rotation of your upper arms, etc. This is your "list." Put *relax my face* on the list for every posture. This way you will be relaxing your face throughout your practice, and by doing so, you will elicit the relaxation in your nervous system and likely carry the habit over to your daily life.

The Chest

Opening the chest through backbends, handstands, and deep twists can release several emotions, including grief, inspiration, joy, compassion, and profound gratitude; this is because the chest is the home of the heart center. Who you are and what your current issues are will determine which emotions you experience. I believe that we should all be doing postures that continually open the chest at least four times per week. If we do not, then we tend to *scab over our emotional wounds*, creating the armor previously mentioned. Deep ocean breathing when the arms are overhead in any posture, including Downward Facing Dog, is beneficial.

The Thighs

The thighs can be silos of anger. Stretching them can release backlogged anger out of the body. Doing so can be very uncomfortable, but afterward you may feel a new sense of buoyancy and optimism. Notice how you avoid stretching your thighs and how agitated a class of students becomes when doing it together. Some of the postures that effectively stretch the thighs include lunges; Kneeling Warrior; backbends such as Bridge, Camel, and Wheel; and Royal Dancer.

The Hips

Sometimes, while opening the hips, particularly in external rotation, people experience waves of sadness. From my study of this, it is my opinion that this particular sadness has a sexual basis dealing with shame or loss of a beloved partner, sometimes even from trauma, particularly from early life. I have observed that women tend to become emotional in hip openers more often than men, whereas men tend to become quite emotional by opening the chest, or, rather, the heart region. Some of the postures that effectively stretch the hips are Pigeon, Cobbler's Pose, squatting, Happy Baby, and Half-Bound Seated Twist. Hip openers that require internal rotation of the femur bones may also elicit an emotional response, but I believe it is less frequent.

The Shoulders and Neck

The archetype of Atlas carrying the world on his shoulders is quite accurate. The shoulders seem to carry what we feel are our emotional burdens, often imposed by outside authority figures or circumstances. So, stress gathers there, making our shoulders and neck stiffen like concrete. Opening the shoulders gives us a feeling of elation and freedom. Common postures where the arms are overhead, including Downward Facing Dog and Warrior I, are beneficial. Other helpful postures include Cow Face Arms with strap, shoulder stand, Royal Dancer, Side Plank Pose, and handstand.

The Throat and Jaw

The front of the throat and jaw are centers of expression or lack thereof. A chronic tight jaw, for example, can be a symptom of unexpressed rage. A dissonant speaking voice or laugh usually reveals an issue with communicating one's emotional life to others. Postures which can be beneficial for this condition are shoulder stand, Heart-Opening

Posture, and Wheel. But no amount of yoga will cure this syndrome without delving sincerely into the breathing practice and committing to honest self-inquiry. You must assess who it is that you feel unexpressed rage toward and attempt to appropriately express it. This may ultimately require a major life change, such as a new career, but the consequences of avoiding the heart of the matter will only be adverse.

Solar Plexus

The solar plexus center is located in the upper belly area, just below the lowest rib and just above the navel. This region is below the heart center and houses different emotions. The solar plexus center is the region where we experience the initial feelings of anger and fear when we feel threatened, which leads to the fight-or-flight response. From the solar plexus the emotions quickly overtake the entire body. Drawing this area open in twists and backbends during posture practice is advised. Another exercise is to lie down onto one's back and then consciously relax this upper-belly area by breathing into it, making the upper belly expand and rise on the inhales and softly fall on the exhales for at least five minutes. This will help to release feelings of anger and fear and restore us to balance.

The Feet

The feet are like portals that bring in energy from the earth and generate energy flow—or the flow of *prana* (life-force energy)—up through the legs and entire body. The feet are like the switchboard of our body and microcosms of our physical health. By opening and strengthening the feet, the entire movement of energy throughout the body is enhanced, along with overall health, and stagnant energy and blood flow released. There is a reason we all like our feet massaged, and it isn't just about sore muscles. Remember that when people die slowly, they generally die from the feet up (i.e., frostbite, diabetes, old age).

The Relationship of Postures to the Body

Backbends
Backbends release vital energy, awakening and stimulating the nervous system. I do not recommend doing strong backbends after sunset, as they will keep you up later into the night. As a rule of thumb, after sunset, only do gentle backbends such as Camel and Cobra. Doing a series of multiple backbends such as Upward Facing Dog and Wheel in the context of a vinyasa class can be done from sunrise throughout the day. Backbends are also chest (or thoracic) openers, emotionally expanding our emotions and keeping them from becoming constrained or submerged.

Forward Bends
Forward bends are calming to the nervous system and bring us to a more internally aware and introspective state. I recommend these at any time of day, but especially for evening practices. On an emotional and mental level they ask us to face ourselves and to become intimate with our own body.

Inversions
Inversions are postures where the heart is held above the head, causing the blood flow to move to the head and brain and away from the feet and legs. Inversions are held for a length of time, anywhere from a few seconds to several minutes.

- *Handstands* are enlivening and promote courage and inspiration.
- *Shoulder stands* are calming to both the nervous system and the body itself, aiding in blood circulation and lowering blood pressure and heart rate. The position of the arms in shoulder stand also stretches the shoulder girdle and the neck muscles, releasing the tension often held there. It also creates what could be called acupressure on a meridian point on the C7 vertebra, which, put simply, stimulates the immune system.

- *Forearm balance* has many of the benefits of handstand, but also challenges the shoulders and chest to open more like it does in Wheel.

- *Headstand* is a unique posture which has many physical benefits that promote longevity and mental clarity, but also, quite interestingly, it also applies acupressure on a significant meridian point called the Du 20 acupuncture point (in traditional Chinese medicine), located at the very crown of the head. Pressure applied there for several minutes is known to calm the spirit, and help to eliminate insomnia.

Getting Started—Advice for Beginners

For your first classes I recommend that you take it easy and allow yourself the immense freedom and joy of being a beginner. Since one of our aims is regenerating health and peace in the body and the mind, setting competitive goals toward astounding flexibility or impressive feats of gymnastics is actually counterproductive. Don't worry at all about how your body looks to you, or how strong or flexible you are (or are not). Instead, aim on practicing with one-pointed focus, breath awareness, and compassion toward yourself and those around you. Do this and you will find that your body will become stronger, more supple, healthier, and radiant without the vanity or sometimes self-loathing that is attached to our idea of "fitness."

The good news is that hatha yoga makes you feel so much better so quickly that it doesn't feel like punishment like so many other exercise regimes, and you will find yourself excited to practice each day. After one month of using a little effort, you will no longer need discipline to go to class. I liken it to a happy dog bringing you its leash, telling you it wants to go on a walk. Often, within a few months, addictions like smoking will naturally drop away as your body, mind, and emotions come into balance with each other.

Postures coupled with conscious breathing can aid us in surrendering our ego and our restless thoughts and lead us into meditation.

Meditation then leads us into an exalted state of an awakened spirit and vibrant health.

Finding a Teacher

Try practicing with virtually every teacher in your area. You will find someone you resonate with—someone who will be just the right person to help you on your journey. A yoga teacher should be knowledgeable, kind, considerate, a great communicator, and show interest in your practice. Avoid yoga teachers who are vain and self-centered. If the teacher isn't kind, move on. If they are not moral, move on. If they miss these two precepts, they are misunderstanding the purpose of yoga.

Also, you should avoid teachers who tend to literally push students deeper in the poses with aggressive hands-on adjustments. Hands-on adjustments are very useful, but only when done gently and mindfully. Most injuries are caused by the ego of the student, pushing themselves too far, and the ego of the teacher, pushing the students beyond their limits. Before class starts, inform any teacher you are working with of any preexisting injuries; this way they can look out for you and perhaps even customize your practice to better help you.

Home Practice/Public Classes

In the beginning, try attending two or three classes a week for about the first nine weeks. After this, slowly build up over several months until you are practicing at least four times a week (if your schedule permits). You will gain momentum from a consistent practice like this, and you will see notable, exponential changes within a relatively short period of time. Some people dedicate six days a week to their practice, which accelerates the transformational process, but if your life does not allow for that kind of time commitment, three or four days a week will be enough to trigger a significant life change.

Although it is good to practice at home too, I highly recommend that you practice under the guidance of a teacher for at least three years before replacing your classes entirely with a home practice.

Begin Before You Begin

Start class as soon as you walk into the yoga center, if not sooner. When you enter the yoga room itself, enter silently, put your mat down without noise, and begin meditating or stretching. Consciously start to calm your mind.

Intention

Remember to set your intention at the beginning of your practice. Intention is extremely powerful, so set your aim high. "All that we are is the result of what we have thought: it is founded on our thoughts, it is made up of our thoughts," stated Siddhartha Gautama, the Buddha. What we attempt in the yoga room is to become better human beings—more openhearted, more focused and patient, and, of course, physically healthy. The yoga room is where we begin to put self-transformative or spiritual concepts into action.

Be Present

I call it "the undiscovered moment." Avoid the trap in your practice of looking ahead for the posture to be over. This is a syndrome that will cause you to look ahead, again and again, never being in the moment. This keeps you forever focusing on a future that never arrives. It never arrives because it cannot, for when the future arrives, it is by nature now the present. This syndrome is not unlike the guinea pig that will eat until it dies, never satisfied. Remember that you are surrounded by friends, people of like mind, who are focused on growth and kindness. They are not judging you; they are wishing you well. They know what it's like to discover the power of yoga. Pay no attention to how you think you appear to others. How do you feel? Again, "Do what you can, with what you have, with where you are."

If you work for seven years to place your foot behind your head in complicated postures, you are going to impress your wife or husband for about five minutes. This would probably be disappointing to you, and you would likely express that. Your husband or wife may then deliver a response such as, "That's great that you can put your foot behind your head, but you know what? You're still mean to me." This is a direct reminder from your spouse that you missed the obvious— that you prioritized incorrectly.

But if, over time, your husband or wife sees that you are becoming happier and kinder since you've been practicing yoga, then you are truly reaping something from your yoga practice that is meaningful and lasting. In this way your practice transforms your family life, your work life, and your spiritual quest. And this is when your spouse may ask you for a schedule of classes, finally interested in trying out yoga for the first time.

Transition Consciously

Practice breath-initiated movement. When you are holding postures and when you are transitioning from one posture to the next, practice breath-initiated movement. This means that the inhale starts slightly before you begin moving, and then you let your movement be led by your breath. For instance, if you waltz with a dance partner, one person has to lead. So, we're going to let the breath lead this waltz.

As Above, So Below

One of the magical gifts of yoga that people find difficult to grasp is that whatever the body/mind applies itself to in order to improve daily practice will be applicable in the outside world as well. When one improves one's attention span in the yoga room, it doesn't stay in the yoga room. It leaves with you and will be applied to anything else you do. When you learn to consciously and deliberately calm your nervous system in your yoga practice, you will find yourself doing the same inner practice throughout your day. As you become more joyful in yoga, you will be more joyful wherever you go. The body begins to be more at ease, storing less negative anxiety and tension; this cumulatively alters one's demeanor to that of a more-relaxed and patient person. The body takes on a new and more natural way of being—more supple, intelligent, and aware.

What if you practice yoga now, but still have anger issues?
There is more than one potential cause for this condition. The first step is to discuss such a problem with your teacher and ask for help. If then after a time there is no improvement, you may want to experiment with changing teachers. If your teacher isn't monitoring your breathing and the balance between strength and surrender in your practice, you may be working too hard, breathing either too aggressively or not deeply enough. It also may be that you are engaging in a competitive/aggressive practice that is antithetical to your purpose. I suggest attending several other classes with different teachers and see if any of them give you feedback on this matter. You may have an entirely different experience. I remember years ago practicing several times with a yoga teacher who was known for teaching very intense power yoga classes, and I liked the teacher personally, but after class I felt off balance and irritable. So, I tried several other teachers and found just the right one for me where I felt wonderful at the end of my practice.

If you feel that you tend toward competition or aggression by nature, I recommend avoiding classes that approach yoga with "attaining" postures as the main focus. Seek out classes that are more holistic and healing.

Don't Compare

Move your focus off your outer body and into your inner body. To really change how we practice, we need to first stop comparing and competing with ourselves and others, and start moving beyond thoughts of how our body looks. We learn instead to keep the mind in the present moment as we practice. We do this by breathing evenly and deeply, moving the sensation of our breath throughout our body. Keep your eyes on your own practice.

Breathe!

Practice your postures with expansive focus on your breath, because the breath in essence melts the ego, like fire melting ice. A powerful breathing practice leads to a life-changing practice. Breathe into your heart center, breathe in light—filling the lungs completely; breathe out the past, that which we no longer need. Inhale as if you were inhaling light; exhale all that is not useful to your life. If you have a spiritual practice, use your own visual image of God or name for God and breathe it in.

Use Yoga Props

Yoga props are incredibly useful and practical. The strap lengthens your reach. The blocks bring the floor up to meet you. Props can make up for your lack of mobility, or support you in more-passive postures. In short, they are used to help you transform your body without injuring it in the process. I've heard the opinion more than once that yoga props are just "crutches" and can and should be done without. I strongly disagree. From personal experience, I can say if one's leg is broken, a crutch is a good idea. Having had several surgeries on my foot and also a broken leg and a broken ankle, I can say that crutches were very useful and necessary for a time. To try and walk without them would have been virtually impossible. After a few weeks of healing, the crutches were laid aside. Similarly, yoga props are used and then eventually set aside, unless the student is dealing with a permanent condition. I don't believe that a crutch should have a negative connotation unless the user of the crutch is a hypochondriac. If you need a prop, use it consciously until you don't need it anymore. If your yoga teacher is critical of props, I suspect that he or she has never had a serious injury before.

Rest

When you begin to feel overwhelmed or fatigued, rather than pushing, rest a few moments. Even horses need to rest. Even machines. We must allow the body to rest, allow our emotions to rest, and the mind to take silence. Allow yourself to move into Child's Pose at least four times in a ninety-minute practice. Learn the difference between an all-out state and a rest state. Many overachievers know only the concept of "all or nothing." Explore the space between zero and ten. Try practicing at level seven, not ten. This will develop sensitivity, patience, and kindness, as well as help you to prevent injuries.

Keep Your Peace

As you leave your mat, keep your peace as long as possible. At the end of class, refrain from jumping up and preparing for sudden impact with the outside world. Do not brace for collision with the stress of the outside world; instead, keep your heart open as long as possible. As you go back into the world, rather than letting others affect you with their stress, you can affect them with your calm, loving peace for as long as possible. As a new student, you will experience perhaps only brief moments of this peace, but eventually, it increases as you learn to begin your practice before you walk into the studio, and to extend it long after you leave. Over the years you broaden these moments between the two points more and more, and your life grows richer and more meaningful.

It is said that eventually, finally, the two ends meet full circle and we live in our practice, our beingness, all of the time. Perpetual mindfulness . . . residing in our heart center. This is the state called *samadhi*.

EXERCISE --

A common question is, How does anyone find time to do yoga?
Try this test:

Add up the average hours you spend on the following or similar activities in a week:

1. Reading newspapers
2. Watching the news on the TV or Internet
3. Watching all other TV and movies
4. Time on social Web sites
5. Reading magazines

6. Chatting on the phone about your problems
7. Working out at a gym
8. Watching sports, talking about sports, reading about sports
9. Shopping as a pastime
10. Doing crossword puzzles, playing video, or other games.

Now, if you omitted some of the hours you spent on these activities, you may find you could easily afford five hours a week for yoga.

I know one woman who is a full-time working mom. This scenario can make it especially difficult to find a window of time to practice, but the woman mentioned goes to her yoga class at 6 AM. Although it's often painful to wake up that early, she says it's easy once she steps outside. Another possibility is to practice with your child(ren). I know many parents who do this, and although your focus may be a little distracted, you can use the situation to practice mindfulness.

-- •

May our practice help to not only heal us, but all those around us and all those we touch in our lives, even those unwilling to heal—may our practice touch them.

Food: Expanding Your Options

When his disciples asked what should we eat, Jesus answered to "be more concerned with what comes out of your mouth than what you put in it, for that is what truly poisons a man."
—Matthew 11

Sometimes when we start thinking about beginning a healthy diet, we look at the list of what not to eat it and it can seem like, "So, what is there left to eat then?" Although most diets wipe out nearly all junk food and fast food, there is so much more good food to be enjoyed. Familiarize yourself with cuisines from Japan, Thailand, Vietnam, Northern China, and Ethiopia, or, even better, explore the eastern Mediterranean diet, which science now touts as the healthiest cuisine of all. This includes Greek, Lebanese, Turkish, Israeli, and other cuisines. They are superior from the standpoint of health and also have an amazing array of tastes.

Our palate adjusts to new tastes. Example: If you diminish your sugar intake, your body will adapt and stop craving it after a little while. The discomfort of change doesn't last long; once you make the changes, you will feel better during the day and sleep better at night. Your vitality will increase, as will your level of inspiration.

Food and Willpower

Health is a little like money: You can pay now or you can pay later. If you pay now with willpower, you will likely not have to pay later with suffering and high medical bills, and the likelihood of living your last years in a convalescent home diminishes greatly. I suggest you do your own research to learn even more. There is so much being discovered every week in the medical community. If you ever find yourself getting lazy and complacent about your eating habits and exercise, go and visit a convalescent home for an hour. It is a strong motivator to take action.

In trying to take positive action, we often get stuck in the swamp of feeling overwhelmed. We look toward the future and feel convinced that the road is too steep to climb. When overwhelmed, the mind freezes in a kind of paralysis and will believe, "It's too big of a change; I just can't do it." In terms of weight loss, if you focus on losing 100 pounds, it can seem just impossible. But you aren't going to lose 100 pounds today, because that *is* impossible—today. You *are* going to lose just a little weight today, maybe a tenth of a pound.

A tried-and-true technique in taking new steps toward renewed health is to stop thinking about changing your future. Release the imagined future. Forget about what you are going to do tomorrow; it doesn't matter, because tomorrow doesn't exist except as a concept when it comes to eating. Tomorrow always arrives as today. Forget the fact that when you look in the mirror you can see the result of overeating from yesterday, because there's absolutely nothing you can do about that. Remember that looking at the future overwhelms your mind with all the work it has to do, and to look at the results of the past may induce self-loathing. All you have power over is this hour; just control yourself this hour. Be balanced in this hour. If you can control your eating this hour, that's all you can do, and that's all you need to do.

This technique applies to more than just weight loss or gain. You can apply it to how you live your life. You can't rectify all of your problems in one day any more than you can lose 100 pounds in a day. This knowledge is the essence of our day-to-day practice. Each day, this is what I can do. Not tomorrow; what can I do *today*? The familiar Alcoholics Anonymous slogan, "One day at a time," is similar in its lesson. Do something that's just a little bit right, a little bit each day. It's the same principle.

EXERCISE 1 --
Remind yourself of these aphorisms throughout the day:
I have the power to control this hour.
By my own hand I have the power to heal this wound.
I am not denying myself _____; I am denying myself sickness and obesity.

EXERCISE 2 --
If you haven't yet gone to see a doctor of traditional Chinese medicine (acupuncturist), make an appointment and get a diagnosis with the most renowned acupuncturist in your area. A good Chinese medical doctor can help you to put together a diet especially tailored to your personal constitution. I highly recommend this.

Also, when it comes to many common internal health problems, it is my opinion that Chinese medicine is far superior to Western medicine because it treats the cause of the symptom. For example, if you can get to an acupuncturist within the first twenty-four hours of experiencing cold symptoms, they can bring the cold to a quick halt, so you will experience a mild cold for two days rather than a harsh cold for two weeks.

Seeing an acupuncturist every two months will create a longer, healthier life, and give you the ability to function in the world with a healthier body for an extended time. And the financial cost? There's almost nothing more expensive than health care for the sick and infirm. The cost to prevent disease is pennies on the dollar. You will save enormous amounts of money over your lifetime.

-- •

The Ritual Before Meals

The taking in of food is something we often take for granted, to the point where we completely forget that the food items, whether animal or vegetable, were recently living beings that now no longer live in order that we may live. We also forget that we live in a society of privilege where we can choose our food from an astounding array of choices in supermarkets, a privilege once enjoyed only by kings. Now it is all too common to use reductive terms for food in an unconscious way of disconnecting from it: A cow becomes a steak, a calf becomes veal, a chicken becomes poultry, etc. We procure our food from neon-lit markets and forget that all of these things exist due to the miracle of creation.

With this in mind, the consuming of food should be done consciously. A meal is an excellent opportunity to practice gratitude, which can be done before we eat. Gratitude does not mean guilt; there is no place for guilt at the table. Rather, it means being thankful for having what our body needs, and having the intent that our actions will be worthy of our food. A meal is an opportunity to remember what we are, our place in the natural world, and our love and gratitude for our fellow beings.

The next time you eat, try taking a few moments of silence before you begin, and you may find that your experience of eating will start to feel more conscious—the way you feel when you do your breathing practice.

EXERCISE --

Write your own words of gratitude or a personal prayer to say before eating a meal. Your words can include the idea of God or not; it is your ritual. The focus is on gratitude.

-- •

Noise

We consume other kinds of food through our other senses. Part of our yoga practice is expanding our awareness and refining our senses with a focus on what is harmonious. Sound plays an important part in this because it so profoundly impacts our nervous systems. Think about how a blaring jackhammer feels in your body as you walk by a construction site.

Once, while in Los Angeles, I was sitting at a sidewalk café and talking with a friend. I became very distracted by the cars and buses roaring by at thirty miles an hour only about fifteen feet away from us. My friend was trying to explain something to me, but two different people at tables nearby were almost shouting into their cell phones. Meanwhile, some pounding disco music was crackling through speakers above us, and at the same time, I could hear a completely different song playing on the radio back in the kitchen. I had to stop and take notice. In the United States, so dedicated to external beauty to the point of dysfunction, so completely absorbed in selling beauty at whatever cost, there seems to be no consciousness whatsoever of the beauty of sounds, music, and, especially, peace and quiet. No wonder our nervous systems are so tightly wound.

Any animal in the world would have run away from the noise that we were expected to not even notice at this restaurant setting. Now then, just add a couple of shots of caffeine and a good traffic jam to this environment, and what do you get? A tight jaw, grinding teeth at night, insomnia, headaches, and occasionally, even road rage.

These are symptoms that yoga teachers see in their students every day in class, in all major cities, worldwide. To help bring harmony into our lives—meaning, first into our nervous systems—sound and noise must be considered an important factor. Noise has tremendous impact on your nervous system. Consider your television; there is a mute button on the remote control, not a cut-image button. When commercials are on, we don't leave the sound up and turn off the image; we do just the opposite, because the sound is more disturbing than the images.

It is helpful to think of sounds as food—as nutrition. They say "You are what you eat"; perhaps it would help us to carefully choose our surroundings and select beautiful sounds and music over noise. If we feed ourselves noise on a regular basis, until we don't even recognize it as noise, how can we expect to quiet the mind?

Our practice in the yoga room is powerful, but we don't have to stop our practice when we walk out of that room. It manifests itself in the choices we make, from our relationships to the music we play, to the cell phone we turn off when we are around other people. It manifests in considering how the actions and sounds we produce will impact other people's nervous systems. The Buddhists call this *being mindful*, and our mothers called it simply being polite and thoughtful. Let's see if we can quiet down our world, in which we've made our homes. The quieter we become, the more likely it is that we'll be able to hear the voice of wisdom within.

SEVEN

Mind, Emotions, Body— Integrating the Three Pillars

In our language and culture, we speak of the mind, body, and emotions as three separate things, but they really are not separate, so ultimately we must approach transformation of the three aspects simultaneously, in a unified way. You can begin this unification each day on your yoga mat.

The first thing is to set your intention for your practice. Your mind is so powerful that it will try and give you what you ask from it. Sometimes we unconsciously practice yoga to escape our troubled lives, but if instead you ask your higher power to help embolden you, you can transform your life instead of trying to avoid it. Feel your mind become a focal point of your highest power. The postures and breath will help you to do this, but your mind must be fully involved. Remember that the you who asks is not your mind, but your higher Self. The Self asks the mind.

Second, focus on your breathing practice. Your breathing should be audible to the person next to you. Inhale more completely, stretching your rib cage from the inside, pausing two seconds, then exhaling completely, pausing two seconds. Keep your breath audible but not harsh. This will reopen the energy around your heart center and allow you to feel your true feelings, as well as your more subtle and intrinsic power. This prompts you to release the past and become fully present. Remember, your happiness is often predicated on the degree to which you are willing to let go of (and not bury) the past. The postures will help you to do this, but your breath must be fully involved as well.

Third, with your intention set and your breath alive, practice your postures with complete awareness. Try to bring your mind into your feet. Breathe through the spaces between your toes. Once you can feel this, do the same with your hands. After you can do both, combine them. Continue this until you are able to be aware of multiple body areas and your breath and the mechanics of the posture all at once. This practice creates awareness and intelligence in the body, along with a keenly aware and calm nervous system.

To review:
- The highest Self sets your intention through the mind.
- The breath transmits your intention into every cell of your body.
- With the intention brought into being by your breath, you embody your highest Self.

When I see my students doing all three of these things, I know they are on the path toward transformation. They tell me that they feel and look better, that they have often made amends with estranged family members, and that they feel more alive and joyful than ever before.

In a way, the more self-centered (not arrogant) you become in your practice, the more selfless you become in the world. The more you work on healing yourself, the kinder and more considerate you are to others. So, you're doing everybody a favor by focusing on yourself for the ninety minutes that you practice. There's no better gift you could give your family than to take this time out of your day to practice yoga with intention, breath, and movement. When you walk out the door from your yoga practice, the internal practice stays with you, and you can cultivate it simply by remembering to do so—by remembering who you are and what you aim for, and what you stand for, always and everywhere.

EIGHT

Having a Code

Every selfish action retards our reaching the goal, and
every unselfish action takes us toward the goal; that is
why the only definition that can be given of morality is
this: That which is selfish is immoral, and that which is
unselfish is moral.

—**Vivekananda**

Ethics as a Science of Behavior

Ethics are a paradigm of living in which you consider the
consequences of your actions on others, and the resulting empowerment
or disempowerment of your highest aim. Ethics begin with restraint—
the ability to not cause negative impact, even if the consequence is not
pleasurable to you personally.

Examples:

- I do not play loud music at my backyard barbecue until
  one in the morning, even though I would like to, because
  my neighbor needs to get up at five in the morning to go to
  work.

- I will not make this business deal for my company, because even though it would make me rich, it would cause my company to destroy the economy of an entire community.

With this type of restraint, we evolve from "I would like to shout at you, but I will restrain myself," to no longer feeling the need to shout in the first place. It is one thing not to say the cruel things you are thinking about someone; it is another not to *think* them.

Showing care, consideration, and effort in your actions—these are symbols of love and respect. Regardless of your good intentions, regardless of your good heart, no one cares what you meant to say or meant to do. Ultimately, it is only by your actions that others determine your love and respect for them. And if your actions are sloppy and selfish, then people will feel disrespected and unloved, and will not trust you. It is that simple. We must never forget this, for it is the principle that shapes all of our relationships, at all times, in all places.

Ethics are partly developed by our environment—our parents, church, etc.—but we all know what *right-action* is. Watch any political campaign and the subject of morals pops its head right out of the sand. Everyone is suddenly an expert on correct behavior. The press provides a constant commentary on the candidate's moral transgressions, even those from decades ago. "Did you know he preaches generosity toward the poor but he lives in a mansion? Did you know he is a womanizer? He said this but did that!" We seem to unconsciously define a person's right to lead society by their ability to be consistent in action, and the ability to keep their word. We all have an innate knowing of what moral or spiritual behavior looks like. How do we know these things? Because we know in ourselves our own light, and we know in ourselves our own darkness.

Most people don't realize that we discuss and contemplate this topic nearly every day. Go to any coffee shop and eavesdrop on the caffeine-fueled conversations around you, and you will hear all about people's lack of, or breaching of, ethics.

"Can you believe he said that to me?"

"She says one thing but then does another behind my back."

"Friends just don't do that to each other. I thought I could trust him."

All of these everyday laments about relationships gone awry are inherently about moral principles; we just don't realize it. Most dramas—on television, in movies, or in our own lives—are really about the consequences of unethical conduct. Ethics are a central part of all our relationships, personal and business, and among our most critical concerns about our government's leaders.

So, let's face it then: To improve all of our relationships, we must have a code of conduct that we willingly choose to follow. Perhaps you follow a code of ethics already, but if you do not, or have become vague about your beliefs, it is time to reassess who you are and what you stand for in this world.

Following a virtuous path not only improves or heals your relationships; it also enables you to break the destructive habits that imprison you. To a degree this occurs naturally from your yoga and breathing practices, even without your intending for it to happen. The detoxifying, purifying, and calming benefits of a yoga practice innately transform much of your behavior as it awakens your conscience. But the shift from selfish or immoral choices to compassionate and kind choices usually will not be completed without some effort. To drop and erase old negative habits, some effort must be made to create and instill new, beneficial habits. One of the chief ways of accomplishing this is by restructuring one's behavior within an ethical code or set of moral precepts. It becomes the basis from which we make our choices, and our choices define our lives.

Sometimes the reason decisions are not clear is because your context and basis for making them isn't clear. Like the Cheshire Cat (in Alice in Wonderland) asked Alice, "Well, where do you want to go? You don't know? Well, then, it really doesn't matter where you go, does it?" If you can't decide between two choices, it's because you are not clear in your motivation. For instance, if you are locked into the path of virtuous livelihood and you're running your business by a code of ethics, it will be easier for you to make choices because you have a code on which to base them. If you have no code, you have no clear way of making a choice. "Will I tell him the truth, or not?" Well, what does your code say? This answer should only take you a few seconds if you have a code that defines your parameters.

If ambivalence is one of your issues, you probably do not have a well-defined code. Defining your code of ethics makes difficult choices a more straightforward and faster process. The next chapter offers an example of what a life code could look like.

The Five Causes (Or Principles of Action)

Who we are speaks louder than what we say.
—Unknown

All great teachers of morality share a similar message, even though it may appear different because it was altered for a particular time, place, and culture. The message is simply this: *Our battles are not fought by challenging others to change their beliefs or behavior; rather, our own personal behavior is all we really have power over in the end.* The presence of a person's ethics, or lack of them, is extremely potent; it has been said that virtue alone is the most meaningful standard by which to distinguish one person from another.

The practice of ethics unites people beyond churches, doctrines, nations, race, or tribe. Universal principles such as the concepts of gratitude, forgiveness, and truth are manifestations of the human heart at its highest vibration. One will find few religious teachings that find fault with these universal principles of loving behavior. These concepts can bring an entire group to the same heart vibration—perhaps someday, the entire world.

If you are a Christian, perhaps you will choose to follow the teachings of Christ. His message was very simple: Love God, love your neighbor as yourself, don't hurt anybody, live extremely simply because possessions bog us down, and allow the power of love and Grace to shine through you. Christ taught us that "The kingdom of God is within." The Buddha's teachings of "Right Living" say essentially the same thing, as do the basic precepts of Islam, or the morals of the Torah, or the Bhagavad Gita, or the Yoga Sutras, etc. The central message of all these teachings is for us to choose a code and follow it with all our hearts.

Following a virtuous path obviously benefits others, but the great secret of ethics is that they also have an ineffably powerful transformative effect on our own being. The following precepts, the Five Causes, are a simple but life-changing code of conduct I have integrated from several traditions.

The Five Causes

1) We practice gratitude daily, remembering that the human heart cannot hold gratitude and negative emotions at the same time. From gratitude, joy and all other virtues are born.

2) We practice forgiving those that have harmed us as a mode of healing ourselves. We reach out to those we have harmed, either personally or by handwritten letter, offering apology and reconciliation.

3) We practice kindness and honesty in word and deed toward all, and especially toward our romantic partner. Kindness and honesty must always remain unified, for one without the other leads to harmful behavior.

4) We practice humility. We never treat any others as servants or beneath us, regardless of their social or economic status. We show respect to all, and are considerate of the consequences of our actions on others.

5) We practice our ethics in our business. Our career is a major forum for our practice of transformation, so we infuse our highest ideals into our work and workplace, always looking for win-win opportunities. We hold firm that the end never justifies the means, and teach our ethics by example.

These precepts promote harmony and reverberate throughout all of our relationships—intimate, business, and casual. How we behave with one another both in and out of the yoga room determines how we affect the world.

Awakening the Conscience

The word *conscience* is becoming archaic in America, and the implications of this are quite visible. Recall the economic crisis we recently experienced in September 2008, with the collapse of Wall Street. This economic collapse was not caused by stupid people. It was caused by well-educated people with high IQs. Most went to the best colleges. What they lacked was ethics. This problem is not confined to America, for we saw similar problems in Europe and Asia. It is not enough to be smart. It is not enough to be well-educated. For a society to thrive, people must live by a code of ethics that they feel in their heart of hearts, as real as their breath. This is called the conscience.

What is the conscience?

The conscience is often defined as "the internal sense of what is right and wrong that governs somebody's thoughts and actions, urging him or her to do right rather than wrong." I think the uniqueness of the conscience is that it is an innate sense of *knowing;* it's not taught, or influenced by others. It is a wisdom that we are born with, and that we all possess. The degree that one follows it may have more to do with one's ability to hear this quiet voice above the roar of one's own tumultuous mind. Our own inner noise often drowns out the inner voice of the conscience.

I believe that through the consistent practices of opening the heart center and quieting the mind, we can begin the natural liberation of one of our highest functions, the *conscience*. Once the conscience is awakened, ethical issues seem to become clearer as a new compassion for our fellow men and women leads us to actions which are kind and just.

Awareness of Time

While the importance of being considerate may seem obvious, there are probably things we all do that are not considerate of others, such as running late. In the busy Western world, "running late" is epidemic. This breaks the precepts of kindness, respect, and honesty. Why honesty, you ask? Because running late as a habit steals time from others. Don't fool yourself; running late causes harm, stress, and sometimes distress to others. You must be aware of how you regulate your time, because your time is your life.

Time = Life span

To control your time is to control your life force.

Dependability is crucial; it is keeping your word, doing what you say you are going to do. If you don't keep your word, people lose respect for you. People respect those who keep their word because this is, unfortunately, a rare quality. A person who is habitually late is often considered unreliable in other ways. Running late is a process of habitually creating chaos and self-induced stress, and to the person waiting for you, your action will usually be perceived as a form of passive aggression. Even if it isn't, it feels that way to others.

For instance, if you make a specific agreement with a friend, let's say a business agreement, and you do not fulfill that agreement, your friend will say to you, "Hey, don't you remember that agreement we made?" They feel confused because they think they must not have understood. And you say, "Oh yes, I'm very sorry," and you give your excuses, and then a short time later, you break the agreement again. What does your friend feel like? Your friend determines that you're insincere and feels disrespected. If you truly did respect your friend, you might have said, "I cannot keep this agreement any longer. I want to change this." But by not fulfilling your agreement, the friend you are letting down feels betrayed, loses respect for you, and the friendship will be over. Breaking agreements more than once destroys relationships, and usually forever. And if you get used to making excuses, it will destroy you a little bit at a time.

EXERCISE --
Time Management
Arrive everywhere ten minutes early. Set your watch for
the exact time; don't play games with yourself by setting
the clock to a fictitious time. (Has it helped thus far?) If
external circumstances cause you to be late, call the person
you're meeting and warn them, even if you will only be five
minutes late.

--- •

Don't Tell Us, Show Us

You yourself are the central avenue for change in this world. Do you
wish for there to be no war? Then eliminate any trace of violence in
yourself. Do you want the world to be more ethical? Then develop a
code of behavior and become an exemplar of that code. Do you want
the world to be more compassionate to the downtrodden? Show us
how it is done. This is the behavior of one who is on the path toward
becoming a being of light. This is the path we are all called to live.

> **What is hateful to thee, do not do unto your neighbor.**
> **This is the whole Torah and the rest is commentary; go**
> **and study it further.**
> **—Hillel (Jewish scholar, 60 BC–AD 10)**

NINE

Ethics at Work

Ambition and Success

W hen Mother Teresa first began working with the poor in New York City, she remarked how the street people there were the poorest she had ever seen. Mother Teresa, who had worked with "the poorest of the poor" in Calcutta, India, and other extremely impoverished cities, found the New Yorkers to be almost hopeless. She said in Calcutta you could save someone merely by feeding him or her, but in New York City, food wasn't what they needed; they were spiritually impoverished and dying for love.

Many people work incredibly hard to accumulate vast amounts of money to buy a really fantastic house and things to put in it, but the tragedy is that they work such long hours, they hardly have time to live in the house because they are always working. Some of these people might as well stay at a hotel for the amount of time they actually dwell in their house, which is used mainly to sleep. A constant state of pushing, grasping, and wanting is not only counterproductive, but also ultimately damaging to our very spirit. Using these aggressive tools for every aspect of our life is like using a hammer on every job, including brushing our teeth. A hammer is a wonderful tool, but as carpenters are known to say, it's important to use the right tool for the job. Remember: If you work like a slave, even if you are a billionaire, you are still a slave.

With a cell phone in one hand and a coffee in the other, urban warriors march through the world of competition and commerce. Their daily struggle is one intense push, and that very intensity can be what gives them a somewhat false sense of importance. We subconsciously ascertain that if it takes Herculean effort, it must by definition be extremely important. We continue using the same tools and methods while hoping for a new result. And when we collapse onto our beds at day's end, exhausted from way too much work and way too little sleep, it can make our excessive drive seem almost epic. Even when our bodies try telling us that we've pushed them too far, we justify our frequent colds, flus, and headaches as acceptable side effects of our sacrifice for our careers. The unspoken Faustian deal we make with ourselves is that by sacrificing health, sleep, and happiness today, we will gain something much more significant tomorrow: power, respect, money, and position.

We convince ourselves that once we achieve these goals, then we can take that long-overdue vacation, then we can sleep, then we can slow down and spend more time with our family, then we can be happy. The problem is that our children don't wait for us; they continue to grow up while we work late, day after day. Our health deteriorates, often manifesting in strange symptoms such as digestive problems, sleep disorders, severe PMS, or skin rashes that we try and make "go away" with medications. And what we all secretly fear is that by the time we get to the top of the ladder, our children will be grown and barely know us, our neglected partners will no longer be interested in us, our health will be ruined, and, most terrifyingly, that our ladder may be leaning against the wrong wall.

Because of this syndrome, many of us are locked up and holding tension in our bodies and nervous systems at the level of combat veterans experiencing post-traumatic stress disorder. This is why we grind our jaws in the night. This is why we awaken at three in the morning, unable to fall back to sleep. So, is working hard bad? On the contrary;

hard work is a virtue, as long as it is part of our transformation and not the avoidance of it.

Unfortunately, when we become obsessed and hyper-goal-oriented, we trade in one set of problems for another. We may achieve our material goals, but move even further away from joy and contentment. The obsessive drive seems to be getting us everything we want except happiness. And again, this is perhaps why some of the highest-selling drugs in America are antidepressants, antianxiety medication, and sleeping pills.

Then why would we take this obsessive drive into our spiritual practice and hope to obtain new results utilizing the same old dysfunctional system? The answer is, we can't. We cannot use the same methods that make us tense and anxious in order to learn to relax and become non-obsessive, and that is the dilemma.

The Full Package

I once had a seventy-three-year-old student—we'll call him Lance—who was a very distinguished and worldly man. He was a prominent film producer and lived in a mansion in the Hollywood Hills. His career was what most would call very successful. He drove a pristine, vintage luxury car, and after two divorces, was still dating models less than half his age. One could say he was still playing the same game he had played for more than fifty years.

At age seventy-three, he was still quite fit and strong, and had become fascinated with yoga. After approaching yoga with SportsLogic for the first few months, he finally came to me one day to say he'd had an epiphany: He had a new perspective not only on his practice, but also on life itself.

He said, "You know, Max, I hate to answer the phone anymore. Every time I pick it up I find out another one of my friends has got cancer. I mean, nearly every two weeks this is happening! You know, they're all rich guys, my age. They've got the full package—the money, the power, the career; they've got the big house and the trophy wife, and they've got the cancer. The full package."

Lance went on to explain his theory: What his friends had cultivated by achieving wealth, power, and luxury was the same thing that made them sick with cancer, leading them to an early death. He was convinced now that the cost of a power- and lust-driven life was . . . life itself.

This syndrome, so common in America, reminds me of the fairy tale, "The Goose that Laid the Golden Egg." As you may recall, this tale ends tragically with a man so greedy that, although the goose made him wealthy with its golden eggs, that still wasn't enough. So he killed and ate the goose, which of course ended his supply of golden eggs. In this example the goose represents our health, and without our health—no more eggs. It is similar to the parable about the farmer who starved his ox.

So should Lance and his friends live in poverty? This is not the message. If you are living your life's work and wealth comes, so be it. You can do much with material wealth for your family, extended family, and beyond, into the greater world. But we must be careful not to pay for wealth with our health.

EXERCISE --
Devote fifteen minutes a day to thinking of ways to help others, act upon these ideas, and watch your life blossom.
-- .

Virtuous Livelihood

Virtuous livelihood is about making a good living,
not a killing.

Virtuous livelihood is inspired by a Buddhist practice based on the concept of loving-kindness and fairness in the workplace—to go about our work and economic life following a code of ethics. It asks each person to determine the virtue of one's own business or career, and then conclude whether one needs to alter it or leave it entirely for a more noble life. It suggests that we ought not to engage in trades or occupations, which, either directly or indirectly, result in harm or deception to others. Extreme examples would include weapons trading, torture, exploiting human beings (such as in human trafficking and prostitution), and the harming of the national good for the benefit of a company. Another example is knowingly damaging ecosystems that would then indirectly harm human beings. This would include causing animal species to become extinct, and even the practice of vivisection.

Kindness is not reserved only for humans, and a virtuous person considers the welfare of all beings. It could be said that the crueler one is to an animal, the less human we become, for it damages human beings to practice inhumane acts. This is not an exhortation of vegetarianism. I have met many kind vegetarians and meat eaters alike. And we know that there have been many venerable saints walking the earth that were vegetarian, and perhaps even more who were not.

If you do choose to eat animals, you can do so consciously. For example, you can conscientiously support meat producers that are ethical and as kind as possible, versus the ubiquitous slaughter factories that have lost all sense of sanity. You might also consider eating only small amounts of meat. Besides the obvious and well-known health benefits, it is now well documented that the current level of livestock on this earth is unsustainable. Raising livestock is one of the biggest causes of land degradation, air and water pollution, and water shortages. And nearly one-fifth of all greenhouse gases are generated by livestock production—more than transportation. Many experts are pleading with the industrial world to return to consuming smaller quantities of meat, as people did before 1900; doing so would help to save our environment from disaster.

When we engage with others through business associations, transactions, or projects, we tend to mistakenly focus almost entirely on the project and the desired result of the business transaction. We become emotionally invested in the outcome of the project and try to manipulate others to achieve that desired outcome. This is business as usual. I feel that our business dealings and projects are really hidden opportunities for improving our personal interactions with others— opportunities for growth in kindness, consideration, and ethics. For when one lives long enough to look back thirty or more years, we realize that what we mainly remember are the personal interactions, for better or worse, not so much the projects. Projects come and go, and fade in importance over time, but remorse over contentious associations or lingering resentments can haunt us for a lifetime.

Perhaps we should look at every interaction in the business world with some reprioritizing of values, and remember that in the end, it is the quality of our relationships that shape our lives, and these relationships that we will remember.

Competition and Power

When a Roman general returned to the great city in triumph, the civic crown of laurel and oak was held above his head. The servant holding the crown was charged to continually repeat to the triumphant general, "Remember, thou art mortal."

COMPETE (v): to strive to gain or win something by defeating or establishing superiority over others who are trying to do the same.

To compete is an accepted trait in most societies, but in the West we have taken this idea to untold extremes. By looking closely at the definition above, one can see clearly that the root of competition is defeating or establishing superiority over others. It is based on animal dominance and not in unity. This mind-set separates us by definition and creates ill will among our fellow man. One may then ask, "But how is one to do business without competing? Without striving to be better than other companies, we will surely fail."

What defines the difference between competing and robust business within virtuous living is partly the intention, and partly the method. The intention: One should aim to deliberately utilize one's resources, including money and time, in ways that are most likely to make life truly better for oneself and others. The method: One should follow a code of ethics such as the Five Causes.

When I was owner/director of Sacred Movement Yoga, our essential mission was to run the center less like a company and more like a church. The difference is this: A church ideally exists to serve its congregation, whereas many companies exist to serve the owners of the company. A church raises the money it needs to pay for rent and repairs, to keep the lights on, and to provide the pastor with a salary to maintain a modest lifestyle. Our yoga school functioned similarly, and it was obvious to others that we did so. We were not a nonprofit—we were a for-profit business—but our policies were more similar to a church than a normal business. Our policies were consistent with the ethics in yoga and therefore drew respect from our community. Our attendance steadily rose and the yoga school was a success: first, in its mission, and second, in business, since we were able to stay open with a steady rise in enrollment.

Once during this time, I had a meeting with the CEO of a large chain of yoga studios. We discussed this very topic. The CEO said, "Even in the yoga world, healthy competition is necessary." My answer to him was, "I disagree. To compete with one another makes us cease to be yogis. I do not mind if you do everything you can, ethically, to bring students into your centers, but where we would fail ethically is if we tried to prevent students from going to another studio, to intentionally attempt to keep another from thriving. If we intentionally try to impair the other, even in business, then we are consciously doing harm, and that breaks the tenets of yoga. Do well, and tell the world of your attributes, but do not try and prevent students from going somewhere else. Do not impair or impede, for this creates enmity and divides us."

How is competition the opposite of yoga? Competition, at its root, is a form of greed—greed to win, and to place oneself before all others.

At its root, greed is fear. That is why this fear-based greed takes the form of aggression, which breaks the foundational precept of yoga: kindness, or non-harming. Competition will often use stealing as a means as well, and this implies deep non-contentment. It is obvious that someone who is truly content would have no need to reach past those around him. Competition breaks three precepts: kindness, honesty (non-stealing), and humility (recognizing the consequences of one's actions on others), and reveals a lack of contentment. Competition is a form of accumulating power for the small self, not the larger Self. It is divisive as opposed to inclusive. Essentially, competition is rooted in the ego, which wants to serve its own aggrandizement as opposed to the greater good of all.

In regard to team sports: I believe they provide good training for young people, and help them to learn self-esteem and cooperation within the context of the team—to put the team before the self. But we must also teach that once we become adults, we no longer play in order to deride and destroy our opponents. The joy is to be found in the game, not in the destruction of another.

In yoga, instead of competing, we try to help each other by being as supportive as we can, treating each other with respect and kindness as we re-create ourselves.

The Ends Do Not Justify the Means

The teachings of the Buddha did not expound, "If you don't get what you want, escalate it." Jesus did not teach, "If you are denied what you want, make as much of an ugly fuss as you can until they give you what you want, so that you will go away." It wasn't Mohammed, Jesus, or the Buddha who originated the saying, "The squeaky wheel gets the grease."

From a spiritual point of view, there is no way to justify pushing, coercing, or intimidating as appropriate behavior. The ends do not justify the means. In an ethical life, the means are as important as the intention and result; they are not separate. Results are in a future that may or may not exist. The present is where we put our means into action.

There are countless people practicing yoga now who are business-people, but many businesspeople and multinational corporations often still misunderstand the value of applying meaningful ethics to business practice. They still follow the ends-justify-the-means mind-set, where-as in yoga and most religions of the world, the means are not separate from the end. Because there is no end, we never really achieve the goal we set for ourselves, and if we do, we quickly assemble a new plan and start all over again. So, 99 percent of our life is spent within a process, not outside of one in a goal-line victory dance. Yoga is a process in which day by day, minute by minute, we are balanced and conscious. We attempt to treat all people as if they are our friends, and then our average day becomes an extraordinary day. Then we achieve our goals of happiness most of the time, rather than a fictitious future success.

The problem goes something like this: David feels that his cause is righteous, just, and based in his faith. He takes action to make positive changes; along the way he sees that he can make better progress if he makes a few minor compromises. So, he does, and then gradually, he makes more and more compromises, believing that the end justifies the means. At some point he does whatever it takes to win, and feels righteous doing so, even while committing hostile or unscrupulous acts to achieve his aim. The person/entity/company he is opposing follows suit in their struggle. And this is the way good people begin practicing evil: They believe they are doing the right thing. The Palestinians and Israelis both believe they are committing violence for the greater good, and for justice. The Chechen rebels and the Russian soldiers both believe their cause is righteous, and both commit atrocities in the name of justice. It is the human condition and has been going on for eons. We need to see with new eyes; let us make the journey worthy of the destination.

Reputation

Our reputation is how others describe our character when we aren't around. It could be said that our reputation is defined by how successfully we manifest our code of ethics.

When I was seventeen years old I was traveling with a friend on my first spiritual pilgrimage. We traveled in an old Toyota Land Cruiser through the Northwest United States, working odd jobs as we went. We were on a quest for living spiritual teachers—living knowledge that went beyond books. We stopped at various churches and ashrams, even a few cults, to see what various teachers had to say. We didn't stay in any one place very long.

We arrived in northern Idaho in February, and traveled to a little logging town where a friend of a friend had invited us to stay at his home. The next day he was giving us a tour of the area, which was mostly farms, when I noticed that many of the farmhouses looked similar. The colors of the paint, the way they were especially well-kept and clean, drew my attention. Our host said they were the homes of Mennonites, a Protestant denomination that emphasized pacifism and simplicity. Some refer to them offhandedly as "less-radical Amish." In the home and at their church, their dress and their buildings were plain, clean, and well groomed. Our host told us, "Everyone likes the Mennonites because they're honest, hardworking, and peaceful. You love to hire a Mennonite because they would never cheat anyone, and will do what they say they will do."

My traveling friend and I decided to go to one of their services the very next day. We arrived at the church in our usual blue jeans and work shirts, sporting long hair and big smiles. We were met by people dressed in a way we had never seen before: The women wore ankle-length dresses and bonnets, and the men, plain, drab suits, short hair, and Abraham Lincoln–style beards. At first they stared at us, dumbfounded. Then the elders of the church greeted us politely and graciously. They went out of their way to make us feel welcome, and, after the somewhat subdued service, the elders and some onlookers gathered around us in the pews to talk about spirituality. They casually asked us to tell them our spiritual views, and then, to our astonishment, they actually listened without interrupting. This was the first time we had ever experienced that in our lives. They then discussed their creed for a few minutes—but in a casual, friendly manner. We left with a very positive and impressed feeling for these people, such that I am writing about them now, thirty-six years later.

This was my first introduction to a community with a sterling moral reputation. Their behavior was legendary to their neighbors, who didn't share many of their religious views. As different as they were in dress, customs, and beliefs, the Mennonites managed to live in harmony with the larger community. Pacifism and keeping one's word carried a powerful reputation that everyone else looked up to.

It is my hope and intention that one day soon, the yoga community will have such an astounding reputation that people will trust us instantly once they discover that we are yogis.

Money

Money is not evil, but it can be made so. Money can be a pure energy if you are rooted in these three principles:

> Your intention is good.
> Your methods of obtaining it are good.
> Your utilization of it is good.

The end result alone is not enough to sanctify your actions in obtaining wealth; the means to the end must also be ethical, fair, and kind.

There are far too many people that behave ruthlessly in the business world, dealing unethically, squeezing their employees, grasping for every last nickel possible at nearly any cost, only to turn around and give large sums of money to charities as tax write-offs, and not from their heart. We see giant corporations do this frequently. In the philosophy of kindness, this is incorrect thinking, and a deep misunderstanding of the principles of life on earth. Your business is your extended family;

treat your family fairly and kindly first; then, if you have extra profits, it would be correct to disperse some to charities.

> **The superior man understands what is right;**
> **the inferior man understands what will sell.**
> **—Confucius**

Our time as students of spirit is not to be focused on how to create excessive monetary wealth, but rather on how to re-create ourselves. Our time is so precious, and our brief time in this incarnation is to be dedicated to our practice, to meditation, to joy, to study, and to service. Money is not evil; it is necessary and not to be demonized, but it is not to be coveted and hoarded either. Mansions, luxury cars, and high society are simply not part of the aim of a seeker, because frankly, we don't have the time. Our time here is much too short to be spent on acquiring things that will be taken away by the angel of death. We might leave our bodies tomorrow. How would you use these last few hours? Remember: Time = Life. Every hour of time spent is an hour of your life spent. It's simply a matter of time management.

If you are enjoying your life and are kind and honest, and you happen to be making a lot of money, too, then you are successful in two ways. I have met many people who are very materially wealthy, and who are also some of the most ethical and exemplary human beings I have ever met. However, if you give up your health and happiness, or the happiness of your family, for money, you have made a bad investment.

Voluntary Simplicity

A few years ago, the World Institute for Development Economics Research reported that 2 percent of adults command more than half the world's wealth, while the bottom 50 percent has just 1 percent. This can be compellingly illustrated by this analogy: If the world's population were reduced to ten people, one person would hold $99 and the remaining nine would share $1.

In America, it's so easy for us to forget how we Americans live in our own utopian bubble. Consider the alarming statistic that less than 20 percent of Americans possess a passport. Of these 20 percent, how many have been to Third World countries? So, then, how many Americans have witnessed firsthand how two-thirds of the world lives? This illuminates so much of our naiveté. And as you know, the majority of Americans watch English-speaking, American-made media, and what we see in the media is mostly created by Americans with American perspectives. As an example, most Americans don't watch movies made in Japan, but the Japanese watch American films. American news coverage is also, of course, heavily American-biased.

We in the United States live on a utopian island where our ideas about money, wealth, and what we are entitled to have become arguably quite skewed. For instance, let's say that you're driving in your car and someone pulls up next to you in what I jokingly refer to as a "Testostorossa" (a ridiculously expensive sports car), and you think to yourself, "Why shouldn't I have that car? There's no reason I shouldn't have a Testostorossa." To us, this kind of thinking is simply being competitive, but to someone in a Third World country, it is so astronomically greedy it's off the scale. Because to someone in a Third World country, simply being born in America means, as a well-traveled friend of mine says, "You've won the lottery."

In other words, if you're born in America, you've been born into an existence where all of your basic needs are virtually guaranteed, even if you're born in a poor area. It means that most likely there will be a roof over your head, there will be a flush toilet, and not only running water, but *hot* running water, and enough food to guarantee survival. It may not be the best-quality food, or not quite enough, but in general, people do not starve to death in the United States. Of course, there are always exceptions. There are hungry people in America, but it's not from a food-supply problem; but an education problem, or a drug addiction problem. It's not like in India where there are enormous amounts of people who eat from garbage piles—not because they have a drinking problem, but because there is no food for them, and no way for them to get it. Or they'll starve their child to make him look more emaciated, so they can call on the compassion of tourists to give him a few cents that will feed the whole family. That scale of hunger and financial despair, this country does not yet know. This is the horn of plenty. To be born here, materially speaking, we have indeed won the lottery.

So, what do we do with this blessed existence? In this nation where we don't have to be thinking about our survival at every moment, like one-third of the rest of the world, we have the opportunity to live simply and put all the rest of our energy into spiritual work, and/or humanitarian work, and/or educating ourselves. But instead, most of us get caught on the treadmill of needing to compete and produce more. Because the bare essentials are no longer enough, psychologically, having only the bare essentials becomes humiliating. When we talk about "going broke," it means maybe we'll have to move out of a house and into a simple apartment. It means maybe we'll have to sell our expensive car and buy an old one. Although we will still have a car, and we'll still have a roof over our head and three meals a day, in America, that's considered failure and humiliation.

Whereas in India or Africa, how many people would love to have an old Impala and live in a simple apartment in America, where they can live and study without being concerned that they or their children are going to starve to death before the next morning? Context is everything. Wisdom requires context, and wisdom requires one to remember global context.

So, fellow lottery winners, one could say we have a responsibility to use our great wealth (even though compared to the person next to you, you may feel like you have no wealth), to be grateful for our great fortune, and then to move forward with the most integrity possible. To lament because God hasn't granted us superstardom is reminiscent of Alexander the Great, who when he was still a boy was lamenting that his father was conquering the whole world and would leave no nations left for him to conquer. How much pity can you feel for that boy?

Mulla Nasrudin was eating a poor man's diet of chickpeas and bread. His neighbor, who also claimed to be a wise man, was living in a grand house and dining on sumptuous meals provided by the emperor himself. His neighbor told Nasrudin, "If only you would learn how to flatter the emperor and be subservient like I do, you would not have to live on chickpeas and bread." Nasrudin replied, "And if only you would learn how to live on chickpeas and bread like I do, you would not have to flatter and be subservient to the emperor."

Imagine a group of people who decide to climb Mount Everest. The extreme journey is meticulously planned, and the climbers learn to work together as a team. Eventually the team gets up to the last base camp, but when it comes time to make the final trek to the summit, only a few have the energy and breath left to make the attempt. At this point the team leader gives the command that all nonessential equipment must be left behind, which includes everything except for a pickax and oxygen masks.

Now, using this as a metaphor for our spiritual final effort to the summit, if the leader of this group tells you to leave everything behind except your pickax and oxygen mask, you leave the stuff behind. The final effort is going to take all of your energy, and then some, and anything extraneous will most likely sabotage your life's work. Therefore, if you get sentimental and overly attached to certain pieces of equipment, you will fail in your quest. You still have the right to bring your extra things—it's not immoral or a sin[1] —it's simply not helpful to your ultimate aim. The mountaineer dragging material possessions behind him will not reach the summit.

Now, if one of the climbers is delusional enough to ignore the advice of the leader, and insists on carrying a bunch of stuff, he may be foolish,

[1] Sin in the New Testament means "to miss the mark" or "to miss the target." It was originally an archery term.

but he doesn't deserve to be stoned to death. His own fate will teach him. Maybe he'll get another chance, but frankly, there is no way to know. It is said, "We are punished by our sins—not for our sins."

I once saw a photograph of a Bhutanese family standing outside their home. They are simple farmers who live in a lovely green mountainous valley. Thirteen people live in this five-room, two-story, barn-like structure. In this photo, they had all their possessions laid out in front of them—mostly things like pots, blankets, and utensils. Propped up on one table was a very old book, obviously a holy book. They were questioned as to what their most prized possession was, and of course, it was this book. I was thinking that for them, once they had enough money to feed their family, then the next money they earned went to that book, the teachings. After survival, there's edification.

But here in the West we tend to accumulate more and more and more things. It may be we are not in actuality addicted to the *things* we accumulate as much as we are to the act of accumulating. Perhaps it is the addiction we hunt, not the prey.

Those of us living in the developed world must begin to differentiate between having enough to be comfortable and having more than we really need. And what *do* we actually need? This is somewhat different for each of us, but a personal code of ethics is a good place to start in creating a context for your decision making.

A friend of mine recently moved his household about a thousand miles across the country. He had reserved a moving van, but once he began packing it, he soon realized that he'd need not only one full-sized eighteen-wheeler, but two of them. They completely filled both of those eighteen-wheelers. My friend didn't see his possessions for about two weeks during the transition. During that time, we had a conversation on the phone where he shared new insight about his belongings. He said, "I have two absolutely full moving vans on the highway somewhere. And if I had to, I couldn't tell you what 90 percent of it is. But then there is still part of me that is convinced I need all of it." He took his realization seriously, and when he and his wife set up their new home, they had a gigantic yard sale.

EXERCISE ---
This exercise is best done when you have been away from home for two weeks or more. The next time you are on a vacation, or traveling away from home for work for two weeks or more, take a little time to write down all of your possessions. It isn't necessary for you to know how many spoons you have (you could just write "tableware"), but list everything you consider to be important. When you return home, walk around your house and storage areas to see how you did. The purpose of this exercise is for you to gain a new understanding of your relationship to your possessions and how you value them. For example, if you didn't remember you owned things that you previously felt were significant, perhaps you might want to reevaluate and reprioritize.

-- •

There is an ancient story of a great sage who lived in the forest with practically no possessions. Once a year the sage would allow people to come to him and he would give teachings. A prince heard of this master and traveled in his palanquin to hear the wise man speak. After the talk was over the prince approached the teacher and said, "I heard you speak and I am so impressed with your words." The sage said nothing, and the rich man went on: "But what deeply impresses me is how you can renounce the world, give up everything, and live in such poverty. I am so deeply puzzled by why such a wise man would live as a renunciate."

The sage looked at him and said, "I am not a renunciate—*you are the renunciate*. I have given up a few paltry items in exchange for bliss. You, on the other hand, have renounced union with the divine for a few paltry items. You are the renunciate."

You can't buy love; you can't buy happiness or inner peace. You can't buy inner freedom. You can be sitting in a very quiet, beautiful, remote place, surrounded by luxury, and still have a lonely silence in your heart and endless negative dialogue in your mind.

EXERCISE --
Ask yourself: What is it that you think you don't have that
you believe money can buy?

-- •

Inspiration into Money

Many of our challenges with money will begin to evaporate when we
become inspired. Remember that *inspire* is Latin, meaning "to breathe
in." It is partly our breathing practice that will change us energetically,
allowing for a more transparent view of the world. Once our breathing
practice comes to life, who and what we are becomes clearer; it is at this
point that we should channel money toward and into things that inspire
us. This can include enjoyable things, but, more significantly, it should
include things that inspire you on a global level. What organizations for
change inspire you? What teachers inspire you? What charities inspire
you? What world leaders encourage you to take a breath of hope?

Donating or investing in these people and endeavors will carry your
inspiration into the world on the material plane. Vote with your money
and heal with your money, and remember the old Dutch saying: We
do not inherit the earth from our ancestors—we borrow it from our
children.

TEN

Avoiding a Near-Life Experience

I have heard of an Eastern Orthodox school where they display a human skull, and on the skull's forehead is written: Oh pilgrim, look well . . . for I was once as you are, and you will be as I am. This and other similar symbols used through the ages are meant not to be morbid, but to remind us to live a fulfilled life—so that we do not avoid death by shrinking from life, ultimately living "small." We must be sure that in our attempt at self-preservation we don't end up having what I call a *near-life experience*.

The Yoga of Dying

Do not fear death. More importantly, do not fear life.

I believe that one cannot really approach a true spiritual life without developing a more harmonious relationship with death. The most obvious reason is that a non-relationship with death causes anxiety, so making peace with it will reduce or eliminate this anxiety.

Death, and the fear of death, are two separate issues or events. Let us begin with fear or anxiety toward death. Fear is related to the emotion and behaviors of escape and avoidance from known threats, whereas anxiety is the result of either unknown threats, or threats that are perceived to be unavoidable. It is likely, then, that it is anxiety we feel toward death, as it is generally an unknown experience, and also an unavoidable one. It could be argued that all anxiety, in its universal context, is generally rooted in fear of death of the body, ego, or the end of conscious existence. Anxiety toward the unknown, at its base, is fear of harm or death. Fear of loss of control is also, at its base, fear of harm or death.

Because of this gnawing anxiety toward death, many—if not most—people respond by going into denial, choosing to live as if physically immortal. This begins at a very young age, sometime during childhood. This of course results in reinforcing a paradigm of illusory existence, as we then make important life choices based on a subconscious belief in physical immortality. This creates a distorted relationship with life, and, deep down inside us, we know it. Then, one day, when the eventuality of death appears before us—either suddenly or as the result of old age—because we have not progressed in our relationship with death since childhood, it can terrify us to our very core. We have the emotional response of a child rather than that of an adult with an adult emotional infrastructure.

To have a healthy relationship with life, we must develop a healthy relationship with the transition process we call death. A person on a transformational and healing path must cease avoiding the meaning of death, and instead bring it into one's innermost contemplation and study. Because of the inevitability of bodily death (as opposed to obliteration of the soul), we know with certainty that we will walk through that door sooner or later, with *later* creeping slowly closer each hour.

You may think, "But why contemplate death? It's depressing!" My answer is, if you think it depressing, then you haven't contemplated it yet. Because death isn't depressing; it is a fact as real as your heartbeat and breath. *It is your reaction to it that defines it as depressive or joyful.* If you were to look again, you might see it in a new way. I believe that the awareness and reconciliation of body-death initiates a much more courageous, vital, and vivid life.

The writer Henry Miller once said, "The ninety-eight years are so much sticks of wood to kindle the fire. It's the fire that counts." This metaphor beautifully relates to the practice and impact of yoga, and truly, all spiritual practices. The practices are tools to help us to transform ourselves. In other words, it's the illumination of the soul that counts, not which practices we use to get there. All physical practices or technologies we use, including the body itself, are temporary technology. It's an organic and powerful technology, but it's what we can take with us after we lose our body that counts.

John Hogan was one of my closest friends in this life, and he was also my yoga student. Many years ago he lost his body without warning from a random act of violence. A stranger struck him down, unprovoked, on the street. A few days later, John was gone. I can still vividly remember all the times I worked with him in my yoga classes—how I helped him with his postures, taught him how to use his body, how to use his breath. Now, his body, or what's left of it, is in a little box, just a handful of ash and little pieces of bone. The body is temporary, like wood. But again, as Henry Miller said, "It's the fire that counts."

I believe that my friend's inner fire, or Soul, still exists. All of the spiritual practices we do have an accumulated energy, which, in the short term, keeps us healthy and vital and increases our happiness, but this energy also travels with us into the next stage of human transmutation. Ultimately our practice is to help us heal and grow, to purify our mind and heart so that we can perceive the God within us, and to prepare for leaving the body behind and transmuting to the next life. That's what counts to me.

We do not know for certain how our soul will transition after the death of our body. We are told different things by different religions, shamans, and mystics. But most of them tell us that the soul is not ultimately bound to the body, and that there is a possibility—if not certainty—that we shall continue to exist beyond the body, and enjoy a far better life than our present one. People who have documented their near-death experiences speak almost universally of the calm and deeply peaceful feelings they experience as they leave their body. And they speak of a guide waiting for them in the light. Some see the guide as a loved one who has already passed; some see a spiritual figure; and many children see their favorite cartoon character or superhero. It seems that the guide is given a form that we understand and will respond to in the most meaningful way. Perhaps in this life we give meaning to forms, and as we transition, we give form to energies, since form is what we are used to.

There is far too much evidence to the contrary for me to believe that the death of our body will be the obliteration of our soul. Having had more than one brush with death myself—meaning, I faced what I believed was certain death within seconds—I have come to fear death less and not more. And from sitting with others as they left their bodies, I have grown ever more certain of a life beyond the body. The more I am exposed to death, the less I fear it.

This mortal existence is indeed short, and the angel of death eventually calls to us from beyond:

> Friend . . . are you ready? Do you understand that your body is but a moment? That nothing you touch with your hands can you bring with you? So then what do you truly own? Whatever is truly yours you are free to bring, and nothing more. So learn, dear friend, that all you possess is in your heart and nowhere else.

Overcoming Fear of Death

If you have ever taken care of someone who is dying, then you know what a precious moment it is. Unfortunately, because people avoid death so ardently, they often don't experience the death process until someone very close to them dies; in other words, until they cannot avoid it. But then, their grief in losing a beloved combined with the fear of their own death heightens the negativity of the experience. What I suggest is that you don't wait for death to claim your loved ones before you introduce yourself to it and sit with the process.

Volunteer to work at a hospice and sit with strangers as they pass away. They will be grateful, and you will learn a great deal. When you sit with someone you are not deeply emotionally connected with, you can witness the event more impartially and without any fear. Then you will become much more comfortable with the process so that when death does claim a loved one, you will not react so strongly, and you will be more available for them as a support system during their passing.

> **When the angel of death approaches, he is terrible . . .**
> **when he reaches you, he is bliss.**
> **—Unknown**

Looking Beyond

As adults, we are often like a toddler in a restaurant who throws a tantrum when his mother takes a saltshaker away from him because he kept pouring salt out on the table. The toddler screams and writhes with anguish over the loss of the saltshaker, as if it were everything to him. We are still a little bit like that, as we often fall apart when what we falsely perceive as "ours" is taken away from us. Remember—nothing outside the heart is ours, which means every material possession we supposedly own, even our own body, is ultimately not ours. It all will be taken away. All of our possessions—our house, our money, our body—all become dust.

So, the sages advise us not to cling to things that will pass as surely as a sunset. Love, yes. But do not grasp and cling. And they teach us to know and trust that we will continue to grow and mature spiritually, so that one day we will look back on ourselves as we are now and see ourselves as we do the toddler with the saltshaker . . . and smile.

EXERCISE --

Heart/Death Meditation
This meditation can be done daily or as needed during difficult times. Try and cultivate a sense of grace and inner power as you use this meditation to shift your perception to what you truly are and are not.

I am in this body but I am not the body. I and the body are separate. The body is mine for only a short time. Even if I live a hundred years more, it will go by like a flash. Everything outside of my heart is not truly mine. I own nothing in this world. Everything I own is contained in my heart. The love I have for others and the love they feel for me is mine. My connection with God is mine. My wisdom is mine. My joy is mine. I breathe into my heart—and breathe out from my heart. May I not waste another moment withholding love.

-- •

A Year to Live

One practice which is extraordinarily helpful as you work to integrate your daily life with knowledge of its imminent end is the "Year to Live" exercise. A Year to Live is an old adage re-illuminated by Stephen Levine in his book, *A Year to Live: How to Live This Year as If It Were Your Last* (1998).

The exercise is simple: Decide how you would live this year if it were your last. At the beginning of each year—on New Year's Day, or perhaps your birthday—make a list of what you would do if you only had one year left to live. What would you focus on? Why? Where would you go? With whom? Why? Who would you assign your material possessions to? Make a legal will for this to happen as you would wish it.

I have done this exercise several times, and I have found that it has accelerated my decision-making process; therefore, I accelerated my life evolution. Procrastination on major decisions came to an end. I made some decisions that I regret, but at least they are now behind me, and I am more on my true path because of those decisions. Before, they loomed as attractive possibilities or fantasies in the potential future. Now, they lay behind me as definite and concrete choices made and then rejected. My life has come more into focus, and I have learned more about who I am in terms of what I want versus what I need, and what I have to offer this world.

Another important and profound part of this exercise is that one year, it will truly be my last year, and I will have lived it well.

EXERCISE --

Use your awareness of this finite existence to ignite you into action. Remember that you are a microcosm of the world. You have the most control and influence over yourself. Search for obvious ways you can replace old habits that do not serve you with ones that do.

Examples:

Every time you read the news, you could instead be reading the words of the greatest souls who have walked this earth.

Every time you do a crossword puzzle you could instead be figuring out how to solve the puzzle of your life.

Every time you study stats on the sports page you could instead be studying something that will help transform your life or the life of someone close to you.

What we spend our time on is where we invest our life force. Time = Life. Never kill time, or you will be, in essence, killing your life. Remember as you transform yourself that you are changing the world.

Grace

Grace is a term frequently heard in yoga classes. It usually refers to the peaceful, fluid movement within the practice of the yoga postures. The yoga postures enacted with grace and with mindful devotion become a moving prayer, and prayer with movement is part of the regimes of many yoga, Sufi, Jewish, and even esoteric Christian schools. (An example is when King David danced before the Ark of the Covenant.)

Grace also denotes a concept of inner grace—a capacity to tolerate and forgive people. These are higher virtues that can be cultivated, particularly through breathing practices and meditation.

Then there is yet another kind of grace, often spelled with a capitol G—what the ancient sages teach is a blessing from a higher source, touching man. This kind of grace usually requires that a person first wishes for it and has opened his or her heart to receive it. In several ancient languages we find that the words *Grace, Baraka, forgiveness, blessing,* and *breath* are virtually synonymous.

PRAYER (N): an act of spiritual communion of one's soul with God, in contemplation, meditation, or in direct address to him/her/it. Prayer can be giving thanks, supplication, love, or confession.

GRACE (N): 1. a capacity to tolerate, accommodate, or forgive people; 2. the infinite love, mercy, favor, and goodwill shown to humankind by God.

To reach toward God is called *prayer*. But the Godhead, whatever it is, is known to sometimes reach back to she who reaches forth, to communicate, and even at times, to intervene. When a person reaches toward God, and then God reaches back toward her or him, that is called Grace.

The form which the Godhead takes is particular to the individual. A German seeker will hear the voice of God in German, while an American child will hear God's voice in English and might see the image of a comic-book hero. The adult Christian will most likely have a vision of Jesus or a patron saint, while a Hindu may see a deity or the face of his/her guru. Your personal experience of Grace will be individualized. Perhaps it is God who adapts the form for us, or perhaps it is we ourselves, unconsciously, who do the selecting. I suspect it is the latter.

It also seems as though the benevolent unseen force reaches out to us less in spoken language and more by means of our unconscious: through dreams, epiphanies, or feelings of sudden knowing. Perhaps we need to expand our definition of communication, and then we may see that we have many communications with God in forms other than words. For example, if a compassionate human wished to befriend a wild animal, she might offer it a bit of food, for the animal will understand nothing of her language. So, perhaps God, like the woman offering food to a wild animal, reaches out to us with gifts as well, but these gifts take many forms. Perhaps a new friendship, perhaps the unexpected and sudden communication with a deceased loved one, and perhaps with our own feet carrying us into a little shop for no apparent reason, where five minutes later we will find a book on a back shelf that will change our life. Perhaps God's motivation is to heal the heart of every individual, and all divine communication is for this primary purpose.

Divine Grace

New Testament Ideas of Grace

The New Testament word that is usually translated as "Grace" is, in Greek, *charis*, which literally means "gift." Jesus told stories to underline that Grace was God's to give, God's sole prerogative, and that it was freely offered.

Grace in Eastern Christianity

In Eastern Christianity, Grace is an energy of God, or a description of how God acts in forgiving and spiritually healing others.

Grace in Sufi Thought

Baraka (or *Barakah*) is an ancient Sufi word meaning the "blessing of God," or a saint, or a sacred place. It is also a term referring to a sense

of divine presence, the breath, wisdom, and/or blessing transmitted
from master to pupil.

Grace in Ancient Aramaic

In Aramaic, the street language in Jerusalem at the time of Jesus,
and the language that Jesus himself spoke, *Baraka* meant "blessings"
(the sort gained by the woman when she touched the hem of Jesus); it
also meant "wind" and "breath."

Grace in Judaism

Berakhah in Judaism is a blessing, usually recited at a specific
moment during a ceremony or other activity.

Grace in Arabic

In Arabic, *Barakah* is a term meaning spiritual wisdom and blessing
transmitted from Allah to any creature he wishes to bestow it upon. It
is also described as "the greater good" derived from any act.

*Seek God within. Clothe him/her however you like. Call
him/her whatever name suits you. But seek. To the sincere
seeker, God answers to all names.*

ELEVEN

Activism

Remember as you transform yourself that you are changing the world.

The next time you hear someone aggravated by politics say, "You want to know what *really* makes me mad?" (radio talk show hosts repeat this mantra numerous times per hour), try answering, "No. What I want to know is what inspires you. I want to know what you think we can do, peacefully, to help improve things. Let's talk about solutions."

Does it help the world to speak about "what really makes you mad"? Are we really doing anything more than complaining? A friend of mine calls it "complaint therapy." But complaint therapy doesn't work because it doesn't change a thing. I know, because I've tried it myself many times. Complaining is usually followed by immediate and prompt inaction.

I would rather hear about ideas that could help the world instead of angry venting about the way things are. A little venting has its place, but too many of us indulge ourselves in it at the expense of everyone around us. As agents of change, it is incumbent upon us to let people know what we are *for*, and not so much what we are against. The great leaders of peaceful reform weren't known for their complaints, but for their inspired ideas and words. Statements of positive ideas inspire people, and inspiration is fuel for positive action.

Activism without Anger

If you watch the news each day you will always find many reasons to become angry. If there isn't an unjust, man-made catastrophe in your home region, the media will find one somewhere else in the world. In this way we could potentially, with justifiable reasons, be perpetually enraged. Many use their rage to propel them into action and activism. But to live perpetually enraged is to sentence oneself to a life of suffering that will spill over and make others suffer as well. This is obviously not a path of peace and spiritual transformation. The opposite but equally soul-killing choice is to make oneself numb to the horrors of the world.

But there is a third choice, and that is *activism without anger*. This method helps to heal the world and ourselves at the same time. I believe that angry activism is one step away from violent activism, and violent activism usually replicates the original problem.

The word *activism* is usually associated with politics, but let us think of the term more broadly. Being an activist only means that we are willing to take action to solve a problem that we consider immoral or inequitable. For instance, charity is activism. In my view, activism is when we take our principles of living beyond ourselves to help others on their path, whether individually or collectively. We take action.

For example, my mother would collect clothes from the local school's lost and found, wash them, do any mending needed, and then ship them as donations to Indian reservations. In this simple way, over the years she supplied thousands of pounds of barely used clothing to impoverished Indian children. She liked sewing and she worked at a school; she put those two things together and took action. Simple. Clear. Effective.

Nearly all of the world's external problems are symptoms of internal problems, inside of you and me. Virtually every political, economic, and environmental crisis we are experiencing today is a symptom of the internal human problems described in this book. They are caused by people lacking ethics, or by people whose limited awareness makes them unconscious of the consequences of their actions. The lack of swift and positive actions for repairing the many crises we are witnessing worldwide is the result of failed leadership—worldwide, leadership uncensored by the people who elected them. We are a population lulled into complacency by the trick of what the Romans called "bread and circuses."

The Roman leaders learned that when the masses were fed and entertained, they tended not to "interfere" in the workings of government. Initiating handouts of bread combined with the spectacles at the coliseums and circuses was a tactic that politicians used to gain popular support, instead of gaining it through sound policy. Today, our version of bread and circuses might be fast food and television.

The grand scale of our problems demands that we not wait for our leaders to solve them. We must take action and realign a misaligned world from the grass roots up. We must—and can—succeed in spite of our leaders, not because of them. Our ethical commitments require that each one of us takes peaceful but definite action to help improve the world we live in. Our ethics do not guide us to become angry and sarcastic, but rather to be activists worthy of following.

When we see war after war exploding across the globe, it can seem that a solution is hopeless, but here's a little-known fact that partially explains why things don't change: The top five nations that sell weapons to other nations, whether legally or indirectly (illegally), are the U.S., China, Russia, the UK, and France. These same five nations are the sole permanent members of the United Nations Security Council. In other words, the same countries proliferating weapons worldwide are in charge of establishing world peace. The foxes rule the henhouse.

As we take peaceful action for change, we can and must guide our leaders to right action, or we can and must peacefully remove them from office and replace them with women and men of honor and wisdom. Every war without exception is a massive failure of leadership. The citizens of nations do not start wars; the leaders of nations do. Ask any baker, farmer, nurse, or mechanic in any country in the world if they want a war, and the answer will always be no. They want to make a living, feed their families, and have peaceful and meaningful lives. They want good health care and the ability to practice their religion without fear of suppression. But their leaders convince them that they must go to war for the good of their families, to protect them from evil, and so the citizens, uneducated about such things, believe them and fall into line.

Over the past two years, I have traveled a great deal as a teacher and speaker. I've traveled throughout North America as well as the Middle East, Europe, and Asia. What I see is that people are the same everywhere I go, with very few differences. There are cultural differences in every country, some admirable and some not so. But wherever I go I find that people are people. They are working too hard and not sleeping well. Many have anxiety about the future. People have had hard childhoods and are now trying to be good parents.

I have found that there are mostly good people everywhere I go. I have been lucky enough to be introduced to different yoga communities during my travels, and I've met kind people who are trying to improve their lives inside and out, and who are working to help others find the light within.

I'm very excited about the fact that yoga is exploding all over the world for so many reasons, not least of which because the world is in a confluence of crisis and yoga just may be one of the great hopes of the future. Yoga is for everyone—all peoples of every economic walk of life and religious persuasion—but for the moment, the majority of people who are practicing yoga across the world are people of the executive class. The good news for the world is that this is the same group of people who have the immediate power to change the world. We are already seeing signs of this in America, where yoga classes are being offered to the staff of the FDA, the World Bank, the FBI, the CIA, and even in the White House. And just recently, a yoga program has been started in the Kremlin.

It's the executive class in this world who has the power, politically and financially, and through yoga, they are finding themselves changing the ways in which they think. I'm not talking about people accepting a doctrine or dogma; it's different from that. It's more a change in their perception. A yoga practitioner is like someone who's fallen in love and now has a different view of the world, as opposed to someone who has had his or her heart broken. It's an internal experience that shifts priorities.

Someone who's fallen in love is more apt to be friendly and kind to the man on the street, or generous to others, whereas someone who's had his or her heart broken doesn't really want to talk to anyone; they often withdraw into their darker emotions, thinking less of others' misfortune and focusing instead on their own.

So, when people practice yoga, they often find that they become more open and kinder to others, and they begin to consider the impact they have on the world. They consider the consequences of their speech, their actions, and their careers. In short, they become more responsible, more accountable. And if these are the people in power, making decisions for the world, this has obvious positive consequences. The world needs to change direction quickly, and these are the people who can do it. You are one of these people.

Every conscious being must take action to help heal the world, but you must be careful not to sacrifice your own practice of transformation to do so. We are much more effective after we have practiced than before. Our role is not to be an activist motivated by rage, but instead by love. Any change we desire in the world must be taught by example first, and by words second. Henry David Thoreau, Mahatma Gandhi, and Dr. Martin Luther King Jr. have all shown us how to take action from outside the system and in a noble and peaceful manner. The method has been laid out well.

MILITANT (ADJ): combative and aggressive in support of a political or social cause, and typically favoring extreme, violent, or confrontational methods.

EXERCISE --

But what can we do? What can I do? Complaining does only two things: It identifies a problem and expresses our displeasure with it. But that is all. So, for example, if we complain about a new governmental policy and then we sit down and watch the game on TV after complaining, what have we accomplished? What will change? We need to express our viewpoint to the people who are in power, not just those who happen to be in the same room. This is what it means to become an activist. Being an activist doesn't mean we need to become radical or militant; rather, it means that we are willing to take action to solve a problem that we consider immoral or inequitable.

Here is a suggestion for a simple process of action:

Day one: After you have identified a problem, feel free to complain about it. For one day. Then that's it—no more complaining.

Day two: Begin formulating some solutions for the problem. Think in four or five stages. Personally/locally, statewide, and nationally or even globally. Never assume that your solutions cannot come into being. Assume that they can. If you are going to assume, you may as well assume the positive.

Day three: Begin taking action. Dedicate yourself to activating one or two of your solutions. For example, send your proposed solutions in written letters to your congresspersons. Put up a Web site. When speaking about the solutions, always present them in a positive and kind tone, and at some point, you will receive help. Someone will hear about your ideas and offer a hand. This is how it begins.

Things to keep in mind:

We need to set an example of what a virtuous and kind activist looks like. How can we expect it of our political leaders if we ourselves are unable to become exemplary human beings?

If you can get something working on a small level, taking it to the next level is not so difficult. But in some cases, starting big is exactly the right way to go. If you have the right connections, you just might be able to move things in a massive way.

Never assume you know a person's motivation, even those of your adversaries. You may disagree with their methods, but don't assume that you know their deepest thoughts, because you don't. Many people have wonderful intentions and are good at heart but make choices based on fear.

Be kind but firm. Gandhi set numerous examples of this. He never backed down but didn't insult or attack. He shamed his enemies only by being an exemplary human being. The British leaders who imprisoned him grew to respect him.

--- •

The Orange Revolution

If your desire is to make quick and massive change peacefully, study the recent Orange Revolution that took place in the Ukraine from late November 2004 to January 2005. In short, it was a series of massive protests and political events in the immediate aftermath of a presidential election that was compromised by corruption, voter intimidation, and electoral fraud. Protesters dressed in orange (their national color) surrounded Kiev, the nation's capital, and demonstrated nonstop for nearly eight weeks. The sheer number of the protesters was impressive, fluctuating in the hundreds of thousands. This unprecedented peaceful revolution was supported by general strikes and acts of civil disobedience nationwide, with the eventual result being the removal of the sitting president and the rightfully elected president being put in power.

In my view, this was one of the most important democratic events in world history, and especially in the last fifty years. It is still shocking to me how poorly the media covered it in the United States. I know few people in America who are aware it even occurred. Yet this was a real-life example of a peaceful revolution that succeeded. It is a model of what can be done on a large scale if driven by ethical principles and behavior.

The more recent Green Revolution in Iran was similar in many ways, but has yet to cause a regime change. History has yet to be written on the results of this courageous movement.

For some of us it is our destiny to lead in the political arena; for others, our path is to make changes in smaller ways. Look at Mother Teresa's path compared with Mahatma Gandhi's. While Mother Teresa was ostensibly apolitical, she was the catalyst of great change in our world. She positively affected the poorest of the poor, but at the same time affected the hearts and consciences of people everywhere. We are not all meant to lead thousands in peaceful demonstrations or to teach about our endangered ecology. Perhaps your path is working with physically handicapped children, or the aged, or maybe you work in a recycling plant. Perhaps you design new ways to utilize the sun to power our infrastructure. Or you may even be the in-house attorney of a giant oil company who is trying his best to steer that company toward a policy of ethics and accountability. Or maybe your way of helping is simply by voting at the booths and with your currency, recycling, living simply, and teaching others to do so by example. All of these roles carry great weight in healing the world.

In the West, many of us have the right to vote. We must use this right. In addition, all of us can vote with our currency—our purchasing power—and we should never forget to consciously do so. And at times it is necessary to surround your nation's capital and peacefully insist that justice prevails. If it is in your means to travel to your nation's capital, then you can stand, literally, for what you believe.

The hopeless person bemoans, "But what can one person do?" The courageous person calls out with an inspired voice, "Let's find out."

EXERCISE --

How does change work? Try finishing this statement: "By this time next year, I would like to be known for helping to create _____."

-- •

**Do not let what you cannot do interfere with
what you can do.**

—John Wooden

Epilogue

The knowledge we need to transform ourselves and our world is available to you. And whether you feel ready or not, the time is now; we have no more time to waste. So hesitate no more. Act now as if God were watching. You will not find a spiritual master that will suggest you play it safe, or a sacred text that advises you to avoid pain at all costs. It is never too late to fulfill your destiny.

At age forty-four, Gandhi was an obscure lawyer. At age thirty-six, Mother Teresa was an unknown nun. Life here is short, so be sure it is not spent, but lived. Do not hesitate. Do not wait to find the perfect mate . . . Do not wait for the perfect time . . . Do not wait for wealth. Act now. Express yourself fully; there is no time to waste.

Take care of your body—keep it vital and nurture it until it expires—but always remember: The last thing our body will be is fertilizer. We are more like fireflies than flesh and bone. What if this was your last year in this body? How many loved ones have you already outlived? Don't you think they believed, like you, that they would live to be very old? Live! Look over your life. What things do you remember? Wonderful meals? Television shows? Endless conversations about relationships? No. All of these are forgotten. We remember when we have taken risks—no matter what the outcome.

As a person takes his final breath, he does not regret so much his actions as his inactions—the missed opportunities. Taking risks defines who we are. Risk breathes life into mere existence. All wisdom resides within; you only need to breathe deeply and listen.

The kingdom of God is within you.
—Jesus of Nazareth

Work out your own salvation. Do not depend on others.
—Buddha

Be spiritual and realize truth for yourself.
—Sri Ramakrishna

About The Author

Innovator, teacher, and author Max Strom is known for inspiring and impacting the lives of his students and has become one of the most respected teachers of personal transformation and yoga worldwide. Due to an ever-increasing demand for his teachings, Mr. Strom travels extensively teaching and lecturing on transformation, spirituality, and yoga.

His teachings are a culmination of his life experience and many years of study. His methods reach beyond the boundaries of simply a practice of yoga postures, and addresses the internal, emotional, and spiritual aspects of our life.

Strom has a unique connection with his students that stems from his own personal journey, his gregarious nature, and distinct integrity. He offers his unique system of transformation as a *Way of Life*, which includes a philosophy of living, self-inquiry, breathing exercises, yoga postures, and meditation, guiding his students to grow into happier, healthier, and empowered human beings.

Born a twelve-pound baby with clubfeet, Max Strom spent much of the first 6 years of his life with his legs confined in plaster casts and braces. After several painful corrective surgeries, he was able to walk fairly well but would always have abnormally shaped feet. This would create physical and emotional challenges for him in many ways. Because he had to learn to endure partial confinement and for a time complete immobility at a very young age, he developed patience, determination and a high tolerance to pain in order to cope with his condition. At fourteen years of age, a personal mystical experience ignited a sudden and ardent desire in him to understand the human condition. Finding little support or guidance in his atheistic household, Max's own passion and intellect guided him and he took it upon himself to read with spiritual voracity any sacred text he could find. By the time he was nineteen, Max had studied Taoism, modern and esoteric Christianity, Sufism, and was practicing meditation and Chi Gong diligently.

After discovering Hatha Yoga he experienced a profound life-change through his practice, and yoga ultimately became for him a system of embodiment that integrated all of his previous physio-theological studies.

Max has now been teaching since 1995 and is recognized by the Yoga Alliance, at their Advanced Teacher Level (ERYT). He has taught tens of thousands of students and trained several hundred teachers. You can see more of his work on his DVDs, *Learn to Breathe, to heal yourself and your relationships, and, Max Strom Yoga - Strength, Grace,* Healing. He also maintains the Website www.maxstrom.com.

Index